1996

University of St. Francis
362.11 M930
Murphy, Terence M.,
Hospital-physician integration

3 0301 00068656 4

W9-ABR-420

HOSPITAL–PHYSICIAN INTEGRATION

Strategies for Success

Terence M. Murphy
and C. Thompson Hardy

LIBRARY
College of St. Francis
JOLIET, ILLINOIS

AHA books are published by American Hospital Publishing, Inc., an American Hospital Association company

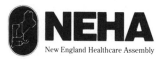

NEHA
New England Healthcare Assembly

This publication is designed to provide accurate and authoritative information in regard to the subject matter covered. It is sold with the understanding that neither the authors nor the publisher is engaged in rendering legal, accounting, or other professional service. If legal advice or other expert assistance is required, the services of a competent professional person should be sought.

The views expressed in this publication are strictly those of the authors and do not necessarily represent official positions of the American Hospital Association.

Library of Congress Cataloging-in-Publication Data

Murphy, Terence M., 1942–
    Hospital–physician integration : strategies for
success / Terence M. Murphy and C. Thompson Hardy.
        p.   cm.
    Includes bibliographical references and index.
    ISBN 1-55648-124-1 (pbk.)
    1. Hospital–physician joint ventures.   2.
Hospital–physician joint ventures – United States – Case
studies.   I. Hardy, C. Thompson.   II. Title.
RA410.58.M87   1994
362.1'1 – dc20   94-27666
                                                                                          CIP

Catalog no. 145159

©1994 by American Hospital Publishing, Inc.,
an American Hospital Association company

All rights reserved. The reproduction or use of this book in any form or in any information storage or retrieval system is forbidden without the express written permission of the publisher.

Printed in the USA

ΛΗΛ is a service mark of the American Hospital Association used under license by American Hospital Publishing, Inc.

Text set in Palatino
3M – 9/94 – 0380

Audrey Kaufman, Acquisitions/Development Editor
Lee Benaka, Production Editor
Peggy DuMais, Production Coordinator
Luke Smith, Cover Designer
Marcia Bottoms, Books Division Assistant Director
Brian Schenk, Books Division Director

G
362.11
M930

Dedication

To Jackie Murphy, Mark Hoyt, and Rob Rosati, who, in very different ways,
made this book possible.

To my father, Clyde Hardy, Jr., whose footsteps I proudly followed into the business
of health care delivery as a group practice manager, consultant,
and, now, author, and whose footsteps no one could fill as a father.

156524

Contents

List of Figures

List of Tables

About the Authors

The authors are cofounders of New Health Management, Inc. (NHM), a Cleveland-based health care consulting firm specializing in designing, implementing, and managing integrated delivery systems. Formerly the Hospital and Physician Services Division of Orion Consulting, Inc., NHM also has an office in New York City. New Health Management, Inc., recently launched a separate division exclusively dedicated to practice management and MSO contract management services.

Terence M. Murphy is president of NHM. Since 1986 Mr. Murphy has consulted almost exclusively to hospitals and large group practices in the areas of hospital–physician integration and MSO development. In 1990 he was one of the founding principals of Cleveland-based Orion Consulting, Inc., prior to which he was the national service director for physician services of the seventh largest consulting and accounting firm in the United States. He writes and speaks regularly for such organizations as the American Hospital Association, the Healthcare Financial Management Association, IBC/Infoline, and the Physician Relations Advisor. Mr. Murphy received an MBA in finance from Cornell University's Johnson School of Management, Ithaca, New York.

C. Thompson Hardy is a director of NHM and specializes in physician group practice formation, PHO and MSO development and operations, practice acquisitions and mergers, integrated delivery systems development, community need assessment, and practice valuation and evaluation. Prior to entering the consulting field, Mr. Hardy spent 20 years in health care management. He served as chief operating officer for a 60-physician group practice and as chief executive officer for a 22-physician multispecialty group practice for the 9 years prior to joining Orion Consulting in 1990. He has written numerous articles and is a frequent speaker at local, regional, and national meetings. Mr. Hardy received his master's degree in hospital administration from the University of Michigan, Ann Arbor.

Preface

Hospital–physician integration activity is sweeping across the United States, creating radical change in the health care field. As of this writing, health care reform is seen by many as an unknown threat looming large on the horizon. However, this threat should be viewed as an opportunity to improve operational performance as well as the quality of services performed. As health care organizations have tried to proactively address reform issues, they have found that an in-depth analysis of options and experiences of providers in their quests for integrative relationships does not exist in health care literature. The trials and tribulations of the organizations that have initiated pioneering hospital–physician integration efforts have remained largely unknown.

The purpose of *Hospital–Physician Integration: Strategies for Success* is to discuss in detail the four major components of hospital–physician integration: processes, structures, business issues, and legal issues. Because the application of the principles of integration is highly dependent on individual circumstances, the second half of this book consists of case studies that address the various aspects of hospital–physician integration. Overall, this book should inform readers on the mechanics and process of creating these hospital–physician relationships, as well as the unique challenges and possible outcomes of such relationships.

Hospital–Physician Integration: Strategies for Success is divided into an introductory chapter and two parts. Chapter 1 introduces industry trends and general issues affecting integration activity. It is intended for readers unfamiliar with health care integration issues, and health care professionals who have researched or attempted integration may wish to skim the chapter. Part One of the book contains the core chapters, which discuss the affiliation process (chapter 2), integration structures and models (chapter 3), basic business issues (chapter 4), and legal issues (chapter 5). Following an introduction to Part Two, seven case studies representing a great diversity of circumstances are detailed.

The emphasis in this book is on highly integrated relationships among hospitals and physicians. Although some of chapter 3 discusses more loosely affiliated relationships such as PHOs, this discussion is provided because loose affiliations are often preludes to a more-integrated model.

The seven case studies in this book were chosen on the basis of a variety of factors. The organization's integration had to be more than one year old and preferably more than three years old. The case studies were chosen to profile a variety of circumstances related to ownership, group versus solo practice, large versus small entities, teaching versus nonteaching entities, and so forth. Finally, selection of case studies depended on the willingness of the organizations to share their good and bad experiences and dedicate the time required to create these case studies. These cases do not present unqualified successes; the successes achieved by these organizations have been borne of insight and experience, and this insight and experience is often the result of past failures.

The authors of this book recognize the magnitude of the challenge facing those attempting hospital–physician integration and hope that this book assists their integration efforts.

Acknowledgments

There are many people who supported us in the development of this book, and we are deeply grateful to all of them for their contributions and support. Specifically, we would like to acknowledge the authors of the case studies, as well as Thomas J. Onusko, Esq., author of chapter 5, who have contributed invaluable experience and insight into hospital–group practice affiliations. We are grateful to these individuals for their time and efforts, as well as the many people in their respective organizations who contributed their knowledge and experience to this book.

In addition to the contributors to this book, we would also like to thank Lou Glaser of the law firm Gardner, Carton, and Douglas, who made significant contributions to the content of chapter 3; Deborah Latimer, who worked with several of the case study authors in editing their chapters; and Dave Roberts, CFP, for his input on retirement plan issues. In addition, we thank Glenn Levy for sharing his experiences and insight.

Our consulting staff contributed their support, opinions, and expertise to the creation of this book. Specifically, we would like to acknowledge the efforts of Jon Scott and Dave White in creating exhibits and conducting extensive research. Thanks also goes to Pat Lord and Lynda Grimm for their insights on physician practice issues and managed care issues, respectively. Immeasurable gratitude goes to Toni Littera, who sacrificed many evening and weekend hours to type our manuscripts, who patiently reminded us of deadlines and helped us to meet them, and who protected our image to our clients and other callers despite the chaos around her.

We are grateful to Audrey Kaufman, our editor at American Hospital Publishing, Inc., who helped us through this experience that taught us that writing and editing a book is a larger job than anyone can anticipate.

Finally, we join Toni Littera in thanking our families who have endured late meals, our extended working hours, and our singular focus on the writing of this book. Without the support of our spouses and children, this book would not have been possible.

Chapter 1
Introduction

Health care providers must change the way they do business. Individual initiative, political clout, astute planning and implementation, and sheer luck can mean the difference between success and failure. The greatest challenge facing health care administrators and physicians lies with developing an effective collaboration. Historically, hospital–physician affiliations have been adversarial in nature. However, to survive in today's health care environment, hospitals and physicians must undergo a major change in attitude and behavior and learn to cooperate and share risk.

This chapter will describe national trends that affect hospital–physician relations, motivations that drive each party to collaborate, obstacles to be overcome to attain a successful collaboration, and the continuum of integration between the two parties. Finally, some basic features of a group practice will be presented.

☐ National Trends

Several national trends dominate health care. These trends, which are interrelated, include the following: competition and the growth of managed care; implementation of federal and state health care reform initiatives; increasing demand for primary care physicians; and the evolution of physician practice from solo to group practice and then to a component of integrated systems.

Competition and the Growth of Managed Care

Excess capacity in the health care industry has created a buyer's market in nonrural areas. Purchasers—both payers and employers—use their clout to negotiate discounts, measure and compare quality and outcomes, and shift risk to providers. As purchasers become more sophisticated, they recognize that medical group practices can provide the best and most cost-effective health care product.[1] The price of services is increasingly based on the marketplace and competition, rather than on historical cost-based approaches.

Managed care, once shunned by physicians, is becoming more acceptable as a means to survive (and thrive) in the current climate. A 1991 American Medical Association study reported that the percentage of physicians likely to contract with preferred provider organizations (PPOs) increased from 56 percent to 69 percent between 1988 and 1991. Similarly, physicians' likelihood to contract with health maintenance organizations (HMOs) increased from 50 percent to 54 percent over the same period.[2] The boost in physician participation in managed care contracting has been fueled in part by higher overhead expenses and declining reimbursement levels. Ironically, this growth in physician acceptance of managed care contracts has also enhanced managed care penetration.

Health Care Reform

In most medium and large markets, the specter of health care reform has stimulated collaboration among providers, involving both vertical and horizontal integration. Health care professionals clearly understand that competitive advantage will be held by organizations that can maintain low costs, document high quality, and promote broadly accessible services. Single, stand-alone health care entities typically have neither the breadth of health care services nor the diversity of geographic access points to attract consumers. Therefore, health care planners and providers are evaluating numerous options for working collaboratively rather than competitively. Internally, health care organizations are striving to provide cost-efficient services, identify outcomes to measure and compare quality, and identify appropriate mechanisms to maximize access.

Price bundling, the ability to assume and manage risk, and "one-stop-shopping" are all competitive advantages. Providers are aligning their structures so as to reconfigure their collective services. The intent is to minimize costs and maximize quality while providing optimal access.

Demand for Primary Care

The physician work force in the United States is, in the opinion of most industry experts, specialist-heavy. Approximately 70 percent of the nation's physicians are classified as specialists, while only 30 percent provide primary care. In most other industrialized countries, this percentage is reversed.

Physician recruiters across the country report demand to be highest for family practice, general internal medicine, and OB/GYN physicians. Yet the percentage of physicians going into primary care, although on the rise, continues to fall short of demand. One reason is that for debt-ridden residents fresh out of medical school, the lower pay for primary care practitioners holds little appeal. Furthermore, primary care practitioners often have higher overhead and are more likely to sacrifice personal time to emergencies and call requirements. Physician payment reform, health care reform, and the overall demand for primary care are likely to improve the circumstances for primary care physicians over time.

Growth of Group Practice

Of all major industry trends, the trend toward group practice is probably the least uniform across the United States. Some areas of the country remain entrenched in the solo practice model while other areas, having embraced group practice long ago, are using mergers to create yet larger group practices and more highly integrated health care models. Increasingly, however, independent solo practice is deemed a financially unsupportable luxury, as demonstrated in figure 1-1.

Current projections are for continued growth in the size of existing group practices, although, according to the AMA, the number of groups is leveling off.[3] The average group size has risen from 6.3 in 1969 to 11.5 in 1991; the number of physicians in group practice has grown from 156,000 in 1988 to 184,000 in 1991. Twenty-five percent of physicians are employees of a group, with no ownership stake.[4] Mergers and affiliations among groups are becoming more prevalent and will likely continue in the foreseeable future.

Figure 1-1. Physicians' Predictions of Growth in Group Practices

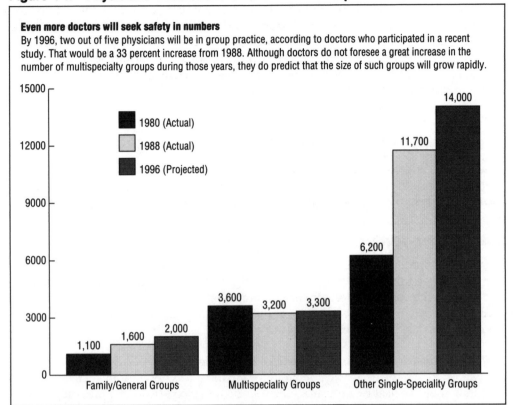

Even more doctors will seek safety in numbers
By 1996, two out of five physicians will be in group practice, according to doctors who participated in a recent study. That would be a 33 percent increase from 1988. Although doctors do not foresee a great increase in the number of multispecialty groups during those years, they do predict that the size of such groups will grow rapidly.

Source: *The Future of Healthcare: Physician and Hospital Relationships*, a study sponsored by Arthur Andersen & Company and the American College of Healthcare Executives. Reprinted with permission of *Medical Economics*, Jan. 20, 1992.

One reason for the favorable projection for group practices is their ability to evaluate and influence physician practice patterns. According to one AMA study, 70 percent of group practices analyze practice patterns, and 38 percent use practice parameters to create practice protocols or conduct peer review.[5] This capability is considered an essential element in future cost-effectiveness and quality of health care delivery.

☐ The Hospital–Physician Relationship Continuum

As previously identified, readiness among health care providers to accept change varies widely across the country. In some markets, providers have moved across a continuum of relationships to create integrated networks. Other parts of the country have little or no experience with capitation or managed care and are very resistant to and threatened by change.

The continuum of relationships among hospitals and physicians begins with *working relationships,* which typically involve collaboration between physicians (often in solo primary care practices) and a hospital. At the other end of the spectrum are *fully integrated systems,* through which physicians, hospitals, and other health care providers coordinate their efforts through sharing of information, risk, and market identity. In between these extremes is *interdependence,* which may be a transitional stage or the ultimate goal of the collaboration. Most of the country is evaluating loose collaborations or fully integrated relationships.

These collaborative relationships (discussed in greater detail in chapter 3) are often dominated by larger entities having greater resources, typically a hospital, health system, or insurance company, but occasionally a larger multispecialty practice. As discussed in later chapters, excessive domination by an entity, especially a nonphysician entity, can lead to problems. Organizations that espouse and practice *true partnership* between clinicians and administrators have shown tremendous success. Typically, the level of provider integration increases with managed care penetration. One could argue as to which is the cause and which is the effect; nonetheless, the correlation between provider integration and managed care penetration is undisputed.

☐ Motivations for Hospital–Physician Collaboration

Aside from the aforementioned national trends that affect health care, both hospitals and physicians are propelled toward closer collaboration by a variety of reasons. The following sections will discuss some of these motivations from both perspectives.

Hospital Perspective

Hospitals are prompted to seek more integrative relationships with physicians for reasons that range from "defensive" survival tactics to "offensive" market share expansion and positioning for health care reform. Purchasers desire integration, which fits the "accountable health plan" component of managed competition. Some hospital motivations are described briefly in the following sections.

Shift from Episodic to Comprehensive Health Management

In acknowledging the decreasing demand for inpatient services and the increasing focus on comprehensive health care management of a population—including preventive health care—hospital administrators are redefining their organizations to become more oriented toward health management. The result of this redefinition is the development of a broader range of services, including outpatient, physician, and home health services, as well as information and management systems to support cost-effective patient care. Because this redefinition requires additional resources and expertise in new areas, hospitals look to collaboration with other providers, thus creating a *vertically integrated system.*

Focus on Primary Care

Hospitals and insurers are focusing a great deal of attention on primary care. In their gatekeeper role, primary care physicians will manage the patients as well as the clinical and economic resources of the organization. As such, these physicians are central to the organization's economic success. For example, the Sisters of Providence Hospital System in Portland, Oregon, a relatively advanced market in terms of provider integration, announced plans to develop group practices with a particular emphasis on primary care. By mid-1993, the physicians' division employed 45 physicians.[6] Similarly, Aetna and other insurers have developed primary care delivery capabilities by acquiring practices and employing physicians.

Better Control of the Market

Hospital administrators view physician collaboration as a means for the hospital to better control its destiny in the marketplace. Studies have shown physician group practice operations to be more cost-effective. A medical outcomes study reported in the *Journal of the American Medical Association* showed specialists and solo practitioners to consume more resources than primary care physicians and physicians in prepaid plans. After adjusting for severity and other factors, researchers found that 7 percent of patients visiting a fee-for-service solo practitioner were hospitalized, compared with only 4 percent of patients seen by physicians in a prepaid multispecialty group practice. According to the research team, the results observed in this study suggest that "physician specialty, organizational structure, and payment methods, acting independently, provide incentives that influence utilization patterns regardless of patient health status."[7] As these results are reinforced by other studies, purchasers will avoid provider networks with a large number of solo practitioners because of perceived and actual higher costs. Thus a hospital with mostly solo practitioners faces a problem. By promoting and investing in group practice models, hospitals can better compete for health care consumers and in turn better control their future marketplace positions.

Easier and Less-Expensive Recruitment

Hospitals also have been motivated by more immediate concerns, one of which is difficulty in physician recruitment in areas dominated by solo practices. Recruitment can be especially problematic in hospitals whose solo practice medical staff are composed mostly of near-retirement senior physicians with long-established practices. Hospital-developed practice sites and practice management are sometimes needed to recruit critically needed physicians in the absence of established group practices.

Hospitals have found it less costly to develop a recruitment package in conjunction with a group practice. Because of the established practice infrastructure and patient drawing ability, income guarantee arrangements with a group practice have been significantly less costly than practice start-up or succession arrangements.[8] Table 1-1 sets forth sample comparative costs for solo practice start-up, purchase and succession of an already-existing practice, and recruitment into an already-existing group.

Physician Perspective

Physicians similarly face a variety of problems in maintaining the status quo. Solo practitioners are stressed out from the growing demands of dual businesses—patient care and business management. From the patient care standpoint, clinical protocols, resource utilization, liability concerns, technological advances in equipment and pharmaceuticals, and changes in technique and clinical relationships will continue to challenge physicians' thinking. From the business standpoint, complex reimbursement regulations, computerization, personnel issues, tax, accounting, and legal issues have multiplied both in number and complexity.

Although group practice physicians struggle with many of the same patient care issues as solo practitioners, their administrative and business concerns are often handled by practice management professionals and/or physicians selected to handle management or board oversight responsibilities. However, groups have additional challenges that often motivate a working relationship with hospitals. These challenges have to do with capital requirements, buy-in requirements, and managed care contracts.

Capital Needs

Unlike a solo practice, a group practice is an ongoing business entity. As such it needs retained earnings and investment. Most groups finance capital acquisitions by reducing physician income in the years of acquisition. Self-funded growth is expensive and creates conflict, especially where senior practitioners in the group do not perceive themselves as benefiting from the longer-term investment. Under typical circumstances, what would be good business decisions, such as growth and normal asset replacement, are often voted down or delayed. In a collaborative relationship, capital can be provided, either through equity or loan, by the hospital partner. Alternatively, the hospital can purchase or otherwise take over the capital-intensive components of the group practice, integrating both entities on a practical level as well as on a contractual level.

Buy-In Requirements

Because capital is invested into the practice, new physicians are required to buy in to the asset value in order to become shareholders. High buy-in amounts can hamper recruitment, especially for primary care recruits with large medical school debts. In a collaborative relationship, capital requirements may be alleviated such that physician buy-in requirements are minimized.

Managed Care Contracts

Smaller groups cannot provide the full continuum of physician services. Therefore, under capitated contracts, they will need to pay out fixed amounts to specialists, and sometimes hospitals, putting the physicians at risk. Actuarial risk of the patient population is also borne by the group. The larger the capitated base of patients, the lower the impact of the aberrant high-cost case to any one physician. Larger entities are better equipped

Table 1-1. Alternate Recruitment Support Scenarios

Scenario 1: Starting a Solo Practice[a]

	Year 0	Year 1	Year 2	Total
Practice set-up costs	$50,000			
Revenues		$100,000	$150,000	
Costs				
Overhead		$100,000	$110,000	
Salary guarantee		$100,000	$100,000	
Profit (loss)	($50,000)	($100,000)	($100,000)	($210,000)

Scenario 2: Purchase and Succession of an Existing Practice

	Year 0	Year 1	Year 2	Total
Practice purchase costs	$150,000[b]			
Revenues		$250,000	$300,000	
Costs				
Overhead		$125,000	$150,000	
Salary guarantee		$100,000	$100,000	
Profit (loss)	($150,000)	$ 25,000	$ 50,000	($75,000)

Scenario 3: Recruitment into an Existing Group

	Year 0	Year 1	Year 2	Total
Start-up costs	0			
Revenues		$150,000	$200,000	
Costs[c]				
Incremental overhead (20 percent)		$ 30,000	$ 40,000	
Buy-in (30 percent)		$ 45,000	$ 55,000	
Salary guarantee		$100,000	$100,000	
Profit (loss)	0	($25,000)	$ 5,000	($20,000)

[a]For illustration purposes, assume the cost of needed equipment, supplies, and leasehold improvements to be $50,000.

[b]For illustration purposes, assume the purchase of a practice earning $300,000 per year from a retiring obstetrics and gynecology practitioner who receives 50 percent of collections ($150,000).

[c]For illustration purposes, assume that the buy-in cost for the new associate is $100,000. To achieve this, the group retains 30 percent of collections (in addition to an overhead charge of 20 percent to cover incremental costs) until the $100,000 buy-in requirement is met.

Note: In all three scenarios, a hospital has agreed to start the physician in practice with a two-year salary and a benefits guarantee of $100,000 annually.

Source: Reprinted with permission from the Aug. 1990 issue of *Healthcare Financial Management*, p. 24. Copyright 1990 by the Healthcare Financial Management Association.

to negotiate with external providers as well as manage a larger capitated patient base. A collaborative relationship allows parties to share risk and usually affords more contracting clout. In addition, a wider range of contracting options is available (for example, price bundling).

Synergy between Hospitals and Physicians

Although the circumstances under which physicians and hospitals are motivated to work together may differ, some common advantages exist for doing so. For example, capital can be raised more readily in a collaborative arrangement used to fund group practice development and/or expansion. Often a dual structure with a professional corporation and a separate capital-raising practice management corporation is created to address the objectives of each party.

Linking of information systems can be mutually advantageous in a number of ways. Physicians can receive timely test results, schedule OR time, and upgrade billing capabilities and electronic claims submission. More efficient physician–hospital interaction reduces hospital costs and patient length of stay. In a fully integrated system, both hospitals and physicians can eliminate duplication of services by combining a patient's medical record, on-line communications between referring physicians, billing, outcomes measurement and reporting, and a variety of other services that eliminate the paper trail and create enormous efficiencies.

Another mutual benefit is the potential to share risk, which over time will be critical as providers seek to optimize resources and align incentives. Other potential benefits are joint planning and strategy development, enhanced management expertise for medical practice development and market penetration, efficiency, reduced conflict over ancillary services, and improved patient satisfaction and clinical services.

☐ Obstacles to Overcome

Both parties must view collaboration as a partnership. Relationships developed with the intent of one party to dominate another are headed for trouble. This point, although obvious, is perhaps the single greatest obstacle to successful collaboration. Following is a discussion of two other obstacles—ignorance with regard to the physician mind-set and conflicting incentives.

Understanding the Physician Mind-Set

Physicians traditionally differ from hospital administrators in their outlook on business operations. For one thing, as entrepreneurs, solo physicians work under shorter, more immediate time frames than hospital administrators. Long-term planning is impractical for solo practitioners, and those who have done so in the past often operated within a group practice setting. Another factor is that additional expenses in a medical practice mean less take-home income for its physicians. In contrast, hospital administrators manage against a budget, which seldom has a direct impact on their salaries.

Physician culture and values are sometimes difficult for nonphysicians to understand. Some specific areas of divergence are discussed below.

Autonomy
As a rule, physicians assume individual autonomy to be an inherent aspect of the practice of medicine. Although this expectation of independence is eroding, the philosophy of autonomy, particularly in aspects relating to patient care, must be incorporated into the planning process.

Patient Advocacy

Due to the complexity of medical care, physicians are trained to interact and coordinate their clinical activities to reach the common goal of successful diagnosis and therapy. As patient advocates, they are naturally suspicious of motivations guided by issues other than patient care. However, to survive in a competitive health care environment, providers must improve the efficiency of health care delivery, which includes efficient resource utilization and stream-lined practice patterns. The key to success may ultimately lie in an organization's ability to incorporate physicians' attitudes with corporate objectives to deliver cost-effective, premium care.

Humanitarian Ideals

Physicians are trained to value humanitarian ideals and thus hold quality of medical care and patient satisfaction as critical aspects of this value system. Part of physician motivation and satisfaction lies with helping those in distress, although this tendency necessarily is tempered by the physician's financial needs.

As organizations plan to integrate physicians into an overall organizational strategy, the thoughtful inclusion of these values can become a key element in the process. This effort can be enhanced by the involvement of a key physician executive as a major player in the process. As more physicians gain training and experience with managing large organizations, they will be ideal candidates to be chief executives of future health care organizations.

Conflicting Incentives

Most hospitals have adjusted to fixed payments for inpatient cases based on diagnosis-related groups (DRGs). If fewer resources are used and if length of stay is shortened, then cost-efficiency per case is enhanced for patient and provider alike. However, from a physician perspective, longer stays mean additional consults and inpatient visits and more revenue under fee-for-service arrangements. Another consideration is physician concern over medical liability issues, which further drive resource utilization.

Without a stake in the hospital's financial performance, a physician will utilize all resources available in the provision of care, regardless of cost. In addition, due to technological advances, physicians have been able to offer more sophisticated services in the office setting, thereby cutting into the hospital's market share and profit from ancillary services.

Past conflicts over these issues have created wounds that may be slow to heal. Under capitation, however, providers are attempting to align incentives to optimize resource use. Both hospitals and physicians' offices will be cost centers, and profits will be enhanced by maximizing the population's health status and minimizing redundant services. Again, this requires a radical change in thinking and the development of cooperative, synergistic working relationships between physicians and hospitals.

☐ Basic Elements of a Group Practice

Before going on to the next chapter, which describes the hospital–group practice affiliation process, readers may benefit from a brief description of the basic elements of a group practice. *Medical group practice* is defined by the Medical Group Management Association as "three or more physicians engaged in the practice of medicine as a legal entity sharing business management, facilities, records and personnel."[9] The four key elements of a group practice are control and ownership, physician compensation, buy-in and payout arrangements, and management.

Control and Ownership

Control and ownership are closely related but distinct issues that are addressed in many different ways. Varying levels of control in a group practice can be held at the board, shareholder, administrator, and medical director level. Ownership, however, by definition must be held by physicians only. Larger group practices can have complicated ownership structures, restrictions, and stipulations, with a separate legal entity (such as a limited partnership or a foundation) sometimes owning practice assets. Ownership may differ between the professional corporation and the asset-bearing entity. (Chapters 3, 4, and 5 discuss the organizational, business, and legal issues related to group practice.)

Physician Compensation

Physician compensation alternatives include straight salary, salary plus bonus, production-based salary, and equal split of profits among other methodologies. Separate compensation allocations may be made for administrative services, seniority, research, and teaching. Managed care compensation may involve profits from a shared risk pool, which would be available based on utilization performance. According to a recent AMA study, more than 40 percent of groups pay physicians a salary or salary and performance-based incentive, and less than 20 percent compensate on a fee-for-service basis.[10]

Buy-In and Payout Arrangements

When a new physician becomes a shareholder in the group, typically after one or two years as a salaried associate, he or she is often required to *buy in* to the group. As a shareholder, the incoming physician will have ownership stake in an asset of significant value. From a practical standpoint, the group name, location, reputation in the community, and group contracts will bestow value to that physician in the form of patient volume. The working capital and capital for the hard assets of the practice were all contributed by prior and existing shareholders.

Conversely, upon retirement the physician is leaving behind an asset of significant value and is entitled to a *payout*. Theoretically, the valuation method should be consistent with that used for the buy-in, but this is not necessarily the case. (Chapter 4 describes valuation methods.)

Management

Larger groups often have professional managers, individuals trained specifically in the management of health care organizations. This is increasingly important in today's health care environment, particularly in the specialized areas of billing and information systems, managed care contracts, and practice expansion, as well as day-to-day administration.

General Advantages of Group Practice

Key advantages of group practice are summarized in figure 1-2. The challenge of the business side of medical practice has grown exponentially over the years. Solo physicians and physicians in small groups spend a great deal of time managing their business rather than treating patients (a phenomenon referred to among physicians as the "hassle factor"). Group practices, on the other hand, typically employ professional managers to run the business. Patients can benefit from the breadth of services available in a larger group practice (for example, physician specialists and diagnostic and treatment services). Many physicians find groups more personally and professionally rewarding. For example, shared call commitments, coverage during vacations, and more predictable hours are among the more immediate physician benefits. Also, payer demands, including quality reporting and cost control, are better addressed through group practice.

On the financing front, the investment requirements of solo medical practice can be onerous, whereas group practice can more readily share capital costs among numerous

Figure 1-2. Group Practice Advantages

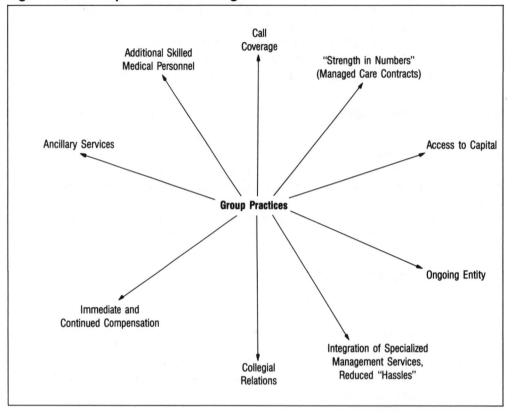

participants. Finally, managed care forces physicians to take risk, and risk is more palatable when spread over a number of individuals.

□ Conclusion

Hospital–physician integration has become a mainstream strategy in most parts of the United States. Figure 1-3 demonstrates the continuum of relationships, from a physician perspective, from solo practice to part of an integrated delivery system. The continuum moves from independence and autonomy to shared autonomy and decision making and ultimately to employed or contracted participation with other physicians in a large, interdependent organization.

Although most health care markets exhibit a combination of stages 1–3 in terms of physician integration, much of the current activity is in the area of stage-3 affiliations. This type of integration is seen by some as an end point in itself, but many others see it as a step in the direction of stage 4, an integrated delivery system. All participants need to understand that the process is founded on relationship building and trust building as much as it is on development of a costly infrastructure and systems. Therefore, many organizations are planning and carefully implementing affiliations one step at a time.

For physicians and hospitals alike, the relationship needs to be one of partnership, which takes time to establish. Some organizations already have spent years developing such a relationship. Others have a longer way to go, a condition that is as much a function of the geographic market as it is of unique organizational culture.

Figure 1-3. Physician Practice Continuum of Relationships

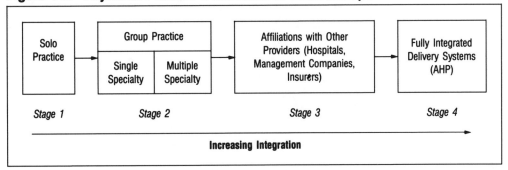

The focus of this book is on the range of relationships described as *physician practice–hospital integration*, wherein some or all aspects of a group practice are functionally a part of the parent hospital organization. Some discussion of less-integrated relationships, such as practice enhancement services and the physician–hospital organization (described in chapter 3), is included as well, because these efforts are often a necessary precursor to greater integration and include many important elements of the process of building trust and integrated delivery capabilities.

References

1. Greenfield, S., and others. Variations in resource utilization among medical specialties and systems of care. *JAMA* 267(12):1630, Mar. 25, 1992.

2. American Medical Association. *Medical Groups in the U.S.: A Survey of Practice Characteristics.* Chicago: AMA, 1993, p. 26.

3. Clements, B. Doctors in groups may lose control with managed care—survey. *American Medical News,* Sept. 7, 1992, p. 18.

4. American Medical Association, p. 16.

5. Clements, p. 17.

6. Cerne, F. Portland, Oregon—The three "C's" shape metropolitan health care market. *Hospitals and Health Networks* (67)12:51, June 20, 1993.

7. Greenfield and others.

8. Murphy, T., and Hallock, D. Group practices tie hospital, physician objectives. *Healthcare Financial Management,* Aug. 1990, pp. 21–29.

9. Library Services, Medical Group Management Association, phone interview by author, Sept. 13, 1993.

10. Clements, p. 17.

Part One

The Issues

Chapter 2
Overview of the Affiliation Process

Although extremely time-consuming and often frustrating, the varied activities related to the collaborative process are key to the success of the affiliation initiative. Without solid and trusting relationships between hospital administrators and physicians, issues and dilemmas that surface during planning and discussion cannot be resolved, and the process cannot be carried through to a successful conclusion. Building trust, however, takes time and dedication on the part of hospital and physician leadership.

The process that leads to successful hospital–physician affiliation varies greatly, depending on individual circumstances and environmental factors. For example, discussions between a hospital and a large group practice would differ significantly from discussions between a hospital and solo practitioners. Also, environmental factors, such as degree of provider competition in a market, strongly influence the course of discussions. In rural and semirural settings, physicians and hospitals work closely together and see their fates as necessarily intertwined. This common-agenda viewpoint is a vast leap from a competitive urban setting, where physicians can evaluate opportunities with a variety of potential hospital partners.

Another important variable is the current and anticipated managed care penetration in the market, a phenomenon that affects the level of motivation and urgency on the part of participants. The case studies in chapters 6 through 12 highlight different processes and results associated with a variety of circumstances. This chapter will discuss how successful collaboration is accomplished in various ways under diverse circumstances. Because most collaborative efforts typically incorporate some aspect of the following six phases, this chapter describes in detail each of these stages of the hospital–physician affiliation process:

1. Preliminary planning (identification of each party's needs)
2. Initial discussions (identification of mutual objectives)
3. Research and detailed planning
4. Reevaluation
5. Negotiation and issues resolution
6. Implementation

All six phases, and their respective participants, are summarized diagrammatically in figure 2-1.

☐ Preliminary Planning

Preliminary planning starts with leaders and stakeholders from each organization (the hospital and the physician group) independently creating a vision statement and strategic plan based on their understanding of their respective needs and circumstances. Participants typically identify some collaborative options, after which potential partner candidates for the collaboration are identified.

The importance of this planning cannot be underestimated. The physicians, in particular, need to stand back from their day-to-day work and be educated as to changes in health care and the potential impact of those changes on their practice. Then, as a group, the physicians need to assess the alternatives and identify a course of action. Without this process, it will be difficult for the physicians to reach consensus, and they will be fragmented in their response to integration activities. Through this assessment

Figure 2-1. Overview of the Affiliation Process

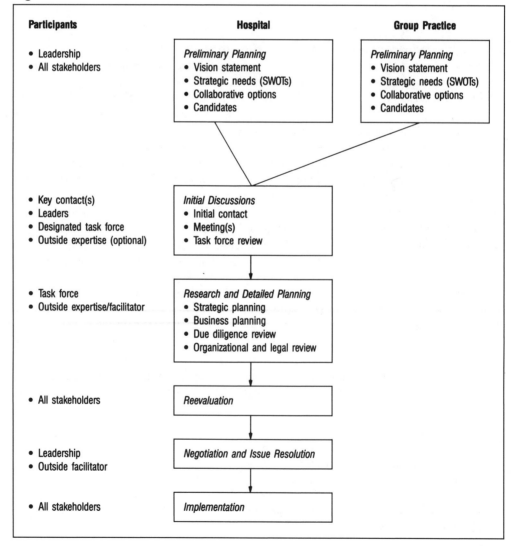

and planning process, physicians need to buy into the concept of change and identify and put their faith in physician leaders (their colleagues) who will carry the effort forward. The subphases of preliminary planning are detailed in the following sections.

Creating a Vision Statement and Identifying Strategies

Before any form of affiliation can take place successfully, planners first must understand what their own needs and circumstances are. These needs and circumstances are defined in terms of each organization's assessment of its strengths, weaknesses, opportunities, and threats—SWOTs—relative to its future viability in the marketplace. (The concept of SWOT analysis is discussed later in this chapter, in the section on research and detailed planning.) Through such candid self-assessment, both the hospital and the physician group delineate a vision statement, taking stock of market forces that influence achievement of that vision. Once this is done, strategies can be identified and prioritized so as to maximize the potential for success. The vision statement needs to identify the importance of hospital–physician collaboration (as appropriate), be compatible with organizational culture, and have the commitment of management and the board.

The importance of a mutually acceptable vision can be observed in all of this book's case studies. In the Monroe Clinic/St. Clare Hospital case study (chapter 12), significant time was devoted to developing a mutual vision for the hospital and the existing multispecialty group practice. In the case of St. Luke's Hospital's OB/GYN group practice (chapter 11), a thorough assessment of the hospital's marketplace strengths and weaknesses and the identification of maternity services as an important component in the hospital's marketing strategy led to the development of a group practice and the recruitment of physicians who shared the hospital's vision. Emphasizing the hospital's vision for delivery of care contributed to the successful recruitment of physicians and development of a hospital-affiliated group. Finally, in the case of the Millard Fillmore Health System (chapter 9), a primary care network was developed to achieve the goals that had been identified in its hospitals' strategic plan—to serve the community and to enhance teaching programs. Figure 9-1 (p. 163), an excerpt from the Millard Fillmore Health System's 1990 strategic plan, presents a vision emphasizing access to care and the development of a primary care network.

The intent of the hospital–physician relationship can be either strategic or tactical. A *strategic collaboration* often requires repositioning the organization to develop an integrated care system. An example of complementary strategic objectives between a hospital and physician group is the following:

Hospital A Objective:	To form vertically integrated delivery system in order to improve cost-effective performance and increase contract and capitated business.
Physician Group A Objective:	To obtain capital resources so as to increase the group's size and its appeal to purchasers and new recruits.

In a *tactical collaboration*, the options typically are more limited and the effort more focused. A tactical collaboration might help the hospital penetrate a specific geographic or clinical market, address a clinical or management weakness, or protect against physician retirement in specific clinical specialties. An example of complementary tactical objectives is as follows:

Hospital B Objective:	To prevent erosion of OB/GYN market share in the east suburban market.
Physician Group B Objective:	To reduce OB/GYN practice management demands and develop a call coverage rotation system.

Even if the immediate motivation for the relationship is tactical, it is extremely important to keep medium-term and long-term strategic motivations in mind. A properly executed collaboration based on tactical objectives can pave the way for and be a tremendous asset in achieving strategic objectives in the future The St. Luke's case study (chapter 11) is a good example of this point.

Once the vision statement, objectives, and strategies identify the need for collaboration, the process can move to the next planning activity. This substep involves looking at the variety of relationship and candidate options to consider.

Assessing Options for the Collaborative Relationship

To achieve a strategic mandate and avoid being sidetracked by personality clashes, conflicting priorities, and other obstacles, leaders and other stakeholders need to develop alternatives for the kinds of relationship and the specific candidates for collaboration. For example, the hospital's first preference may be to affiliate with a dominant 10-physician primary care group. However, because of past personality conflicts, the group may have no interest in getting involved in an integrated relationship with the hospital. Therefore, alternatives, such as other group practices or physicians willing to develop a new group practice, should be identified as secondary options.

The nature of the hospital–physician relationship ultimately is a product of several factors, among them the needs of the constituent organizations, the environment, and the climate in which the negotiation process was conducted. However, based on the planning accomplished thus far, at least a general sense of the type of collaborative relationship should be established. Relationships range from the benign, including practice enhancement seminars and physician recruitment assistance, to the complete organizational and financial integration of group practice and hospital. In between these two extremes is where most of the market activity around the country is focused, represented by labels such as *physician–hospital organizations* (PHOs), *management service organizations* (MSOs), *group practice without walls* (GPWW), *foundation models, captive professional corporations* (PCs), and so on. Figure 2-2 shows these relationships on a continuum from least integrated to most integrated. (Chapter 3 describes these relationships in greater detail.)

Market forces appear to be driving providers to more fully integrated models. However, rather than leaping hastily into the more integrated side of the continuum, it may make more sense for an organization with little or no experience in this area to consider a gradual move into collaborative relationships. This might be done by initially developing a managed care contracting entity such as a PHO, or by developing practice management capability (MSOs). Both options offer collaborating practices a common denominator and a foundation for future practice integration.

On the other hand, at least three factors might argue for moving more quickly toward an integrated relationship. These factors include (1) pressures of market dynamics and purchaser demands, (2) current or anticipated alternatives available to physicians, and (3) the potential that the intermediate collaborative relationship can be counterproductive to long-term goals—a dead end resulting in loss of physician interest, valuable time, and trust.

The gradual approach appears to be advantageous in most cases because it takes time to restructure the organization and initiate new business ventures. Two realities support this approach. First, in the business of medical practice management and clinical care, the level of sophistication required for large-scale practice management is often underestimated by hospital administrators. This business segment is very different from the business of managing a hospital, and it demands an investment in professionals experienced in practice management. Overlooking this issue can lead to failure of the collaborative venture.

Second, health care providers are subjected to a 180-degree change in the way they approach the economics of health care when they go from fee-for-service to capitation.

Figure 2-2. Continuum of Hospital–Physician Integration

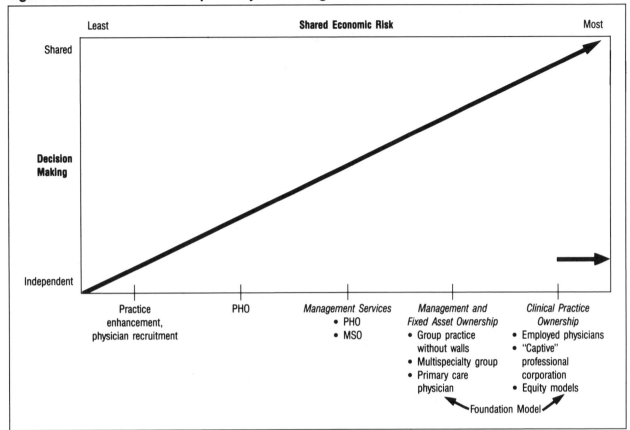

Under capitation, facilities, product lines, and staff (including physicians) are all categorized as overhead expense. Because the organization is paid up front, the economic incentive is to incur the least cost possible in providing care to the designated population. Emphasis is on disease prevention, health maintenance and promotion programs, early detection, and less-costly and less-invasive treatments.

In implementing these changes, it takes time to build physician trust. Although investment in experienced personnel and sophisticated billing and information systems can speed progress, there is no shortcut to gaining trust.

Only through sober assessment of its capabilities and position regarding the key issues of practice management, managed care, and physician trust can each organization decide how fast to move toward full integration. To evaluate each relationship option at this early stage, it is useful to answer the following questions:

- Does the option accomplish the strategic need?
- Does it significantly compromise other strategic mandates?
- Is it consistent with, and can it be built upon in order to achieve, longer-term goals?
- Is it practical?
- Can it be communicated?
- Does it constitute too much change, too fast?
- Does it impose too little change, too slow?

Without close attention to organizational needs, environmental factors, and the negotiation process itself, strategies for developing appropriate relationship options and range of integration can be compromised.

Candidates for Collaboration

After planners have weighed various collaborative options, specific candidates should be considered for the relationship. Again, key questions need to be asked, including:

- Do we understand the needs of the other party? (The answer here must be carefully considered. Many potential relationships never get under way because one party does not clearly understand the other's needs, as discussed earlier.)
- Is there a trusting relationship, or at least the absence of "bad blood" between candidates and the hospital?
- Is there good leadership structure in the candidates' organizations?
- What do we have that they could benefit from, and vice versa?
- What alternatives exist to the partner under consideration?

Because formal collaboration is typically a long-term relationship and the physician participants at the outset will form the foundation for these relationships, it is important to work with the right physicians or, perhaps more important, not to work with the wrong physicians from a managed care standpoint. Therefore, at the outset the health care organization should seek to understand the relative performance of physician candidates from a managed care perspective, that is, evaluating issues such as physician cost-efficiency and quality. In this and other ways, the organization seeking to collaborate needs to look beyond the actual affiliation negotiation to the long-term strategy. Ultimate success will depend on the competitiveness of the combined entity in a managed care environment. Clearly it is more difficult, although not impossible, to change physician behavior after the relationship is established than to involve the right physician(s) from the start.

After considering candidate options, a "Plan A" strategy should be developed that identifies the preferred partner(s) for the affiliation. The candidate's leadership structure, group culture, managed care involvement, and any unique circumstances need to be understood by using all resources available. Resources can include discussions with hospital personnel and/or physicians familiar with the group, hospital records on physician practice patterns, and managed provider panels. "Plan B" and "Plan C" physician and/or group alternatives should be defined as well, should Plan A fail.

It is a good idea to set a general timetable for the discussion and negotiation process. In the event the Plan A choice does not appear viable, mutual agreement should dictate that Plans B and C be pursued at once, assuming that a collaborative relationship is a strategic mandate for the organization. A word of caution: In these fast-paced times, affiliation discussions have a way of falling apart and then reemerging. The hospital would be well advised to help Plan A participants understand and accept its need to pursue alternatives should the physician(s) be unable or unwilling to move forward with collaboration. Making this clear leaves the door open for both parties to continue to pursue their best interests, yet return to the negotiation table at a future opportunity without negative baggage.

☐ Initial Discussions

The initial discussion stage includes two components. The first is an informal contact that gets the message across to the physicians about the hospital's interest in cultivating a relationship. The second is a formal meeting during which the parties listen to each other and gain some understanding of their respective concerns. As mentioned earlier, the entire process of building a hospital–physician affiliation rests on building trust. Once established, this trust is fragile. Months, even years, of effort can be sidetracked by an ill-conceived or miscalculated action. The two components of initial discussions, informal contact and informal meeting, are discussed in detail below.

The Initial Contact

The message conveyed during the initial contact should be neither too strong nor too weak. Too strong a message, such as the absolute resolution of the hospital to "own and control medical practices," can put physicians on the defensive, send them looking for alternative partners, or stir rampant rumors throughout the medical staff. On the other hand, too weak a message can understate an organization's commitment to change, create ambiguity, confuse the potential collaborator, or slow down the process. An appropriate message expresses a motivation to change based on a clear understanding of current short-comings and future needs, an openness to discuss options, and a commitment to develop an organizational advantage within a defined time frame.

The method and vehicle for delivery of the initial message depends on the circumstances and the nature of the prospective relationships. Generally, however, the means should be an informal discussion between a top hospital administrator and a key physician leader of the target group. This preliminary contact should result in a mutual interest to gain a more thorough understanding of one another's objectives, needs, and "sacred ground" criteria—that is, those elements considered an absolute must or potential deal-breaker. Overall, this discussion should be casual and, to the extent possible, confidential.

The Formal Meeting

The second meeting is more formal, an opportunity for the parties to bring to the table their thoughts and concerns regarding a potential relationship. The specific goals of this meeting are to gain a mutual understanding of present circumstances and the parties' vision for the future. It is important for hospital administrators and group physician leaders to view the prospective collaboration through one another's eyes.

Participants should use this more formalized forum to evaluate whether the parties need to be educated regarding evolution and change within the health care industry. Education can be a common denominator that enlightens participants on a common set of market realities—for example, changing purchaser demands. Physicians and hospitals do not experience the same health care marketplace realities; physicians may be less attuned to macro trends and issues, although they do have frontline information as to current marketplace events. Hospital administrators need to be educated on the physicians' experience and perspective as well. For example, hospital management must recognize physicians' expectations of and need for rapid response from the operations of a practice. Physicians, faced with a large number of patients demanding immediate results for their problems, must have responsive support in their practice. This work atmosphere, combined with the sole proprietorship of many practices acquired by hospitals (where physicians controlled the demand and utilization of information, resources, and all other aspects of the practices), creates the need for an adjustment from traditional hospital management approaches to patient service operations. This willingness to listen to each other further builds understanding and mutual trust.

Consideration should be given to involving an objective outside facilitator who can help keep the discussions moving forward in a productive manner. Past and current experiences, even if relevant, can sidetrack the discussion. An outside facilitator can be beneficial if he or she is familiar with this "baggage" and therefore able to keep the discussion on track.

These meetings often result in the definition of common ground and positive interest for more formal discussions. At that point, an exploratory task force made up of representatives from both organizations should be created, particularly for discussions that involve multiple physicians or group practices.

Exploratory Task Force

The exploratory task force is charged with investigating the potential of an integrated relationship. The ideal size for this group is five or six, with three physician participants and two or three hospital participants. It is particularly important that, from the physician standpoint, task force participants be well respected as "opinion leaders" among their peers and able to represent the needs and objectives of their constituencies.

The task force usually engages in a series of meetings that combine education and open discussion. Often participants, particularly the physicians, approach the collaboration discussions with a degree of trepidation. Given the history of hospital–physician relationships, this is understandable. However, as the market becomes more competitive and the economic climate continues to force hospitals and physicians to work together constructively for mutual benefit and survival, timing becomes increasingly important. It is simply unwise for either party to invest significant time in an integrated relationship, only to have the affiliation fail in future years because the terms of the arrangement favored one party over the other beyond what is acceptable. More and more, affiliation discussants are recognizing that win–lose scenarios, where one party benefits at the expense of another, deteriorate into lose–lose scenarios.

The ultimate goal of the task force, then, is to identify a common strategic vision and advantages that mutually benefit all parties concerned—that is, to arrive at a win–win scenario. A win–win scenario is important because, typically, neither party can afford the fallout and setbacks caused by a failed relationship. The common vision (which should be consistent with the visions of the respective entities established prior to the task force meetings) must encompass the needs and objectives of both parties. Two natural spin-offs of creating the vision statement are identification of problems as well as subsequent steps in the discussion process.

Problem Identification

As a result of task force meetings and discussions, various issues and problem areas can be identified. Some of these issues (for example, managed care contracting requirements or legal and tax issues) may be addressed through research. Others (such as marketplace competition) may be reidentified as opportunities and addressed by financial or market analysis. Certain other issues—perhaps ancillary service expansion or ownership—may represent negotiation points or "deal-breakers." By categorizing issues in this manner, the task force determines when and how they are best handled.

Subsequent Steps in the Process

The next steps vary depending on the organization's circumstances and can include educational programs, development and review of relationship options, financial research, and/or consensus building. Most important, the task force makes a recommendation back to its constituencies as to the potential for collaborative relationship. If the consensus is to move forward, the discussion moves into a research and detailed planning component. The task force should determine who will bear costs related to any needed outside assistance and, in conjunction with leadership of the represented entities, assign responsibilities and time frames for these efforts.

An option at this point is to develop an "informal formalization" of progress to date by outlining the common vision and objectives in a letter of intent. A *letter of intent* is a document that demonstrates good faith on the part of both parties and a commitment to serious assessment of the opportunity to affiliate. This document is important because the ensuing financial, legal, and business research will likely require investment in outside expertise.

☐ Research and Detailed Planning

The research and detailed planning phase is an iterative process designed so that both parties work together to investigate the comparative implications of relationship alternatives. Key participants are the task force members, unless otherwise indicated. The desired outcome of this stage of the discussion process is a firm, carefully considered consensus on the nature of the potential business relationship, arrived at through SWOT assessment, evaluation of relationship alternatives, review of legal issues, and consideration of financial implications. Although key issues such as physician compensation, payments for asset acquisition, and details of decision making and control remain to be negotiated, the basic parameters of the arrangement need to be established and agreed on first. The research and detailed planning phase encompasses a number of discrete activities, among them strategic planning, business planning, due diligence, and organizational and legal assessment.

Strategic Planning

Based on preliminary task force feedback, particularly from physicians, it may be advisable to conduct a combined strategic planning retreat. This is an opportunity for the respective parties to ratify or modify results of task force findings and to move the planning process a step forward. The purpose and results of the strategic planning effort can include the following:

- Definition or refinement of the common vision
- Identification of key issues to be resolved
- Development of consensus by virtue of full participation of physicians and hospital administration
- Building of a sense of common purpose and commitment
- Identification of potential leaders and key participants

The result of the strategic planning effort should be an organizationwide "stamp of approval" for all affiliation efforts to date, thus building momentum to move forward. At this juncture, an outside facilitator is a likely requirement. In addition to facilitation skills, this individual brings an element of neutrality to the combined objective while reinforcing commitment to the overall effort.

An effective strategic planning session typically involves some upfront research on the part of the facilitator. He or she may initiate personal interviews with key participants in the process that are designed to gain an understanding of the cultures, specific needs, and concerns of the respective parties. In addition, the facilitator should conduct some basic market research, including an examination of competitors, payer trends, geographic issues, and recent market developments. Through the use of these two tools—interviews and market research—the facilitator can develop a preliminary profile of the hospital and physician group's *strengths, weaknesses, opportunities, and threats* (SWOTs).

Organizational *strengths and weaknesses* relate to internal capabilities, demonstrated performance, or other features inherent to the organization. Examples include location; reputation; historical experience of personnel, product, or service performance; financial performance; assets; and specific product lines. *Opportunities and threats* typically are circumstances that can enable the organization to attain positive or negative outcomes. Examples include health care reform, competitor activity, new markets, new product lines, operational changes, and pricing.

Usually the retreat lasts a full day and should be conducted off-site to ensure a minimum of interruptions. Commonly, the retreat agenda includes introductory remarks from leaders of both organizations, a review of progress to date, presentation and elaboration on the SWOT analysis of both organizations, definition (or redefinition) of common vision and objectives, and delineation of issues to be addressed. Opposing and challenging viewpoints should be encouraged; however, the facilitator must be alert to unproductive avenues of discussion and keep the conversation on track.

Within a week after the strategic planning session, the results should be compiled and submitted in draft form to leaders for review and comment. This is a critical juncture, for word of the planning effort will have spread by now. Also, participants will have thought about the discussion and given feedback to the designated leadership as to any major issues and problems. This juncture is the first major reality test for the future of the integrated relationship. If no major problems are apparent, both parties should be comfortable in moving forward to the next step, which includes two concurrent efforts: development of a general business plan and due diligence. If problems surface at this point, then either the common vision needs to be reevaluated or other alternatives need to be considered to achieve common objectives. In many cases, further education is needed to understand industry trends and available alternatives.

Business Planning

Broadly stated, the purpose of this step is to evaluate the anticipated performance of the respective entities under the new relationship and to arrive at a consensus regarding business, legal, and structural options for the relationship. The same task force is involved, perhaps with a few additions, although a maximum of eight participants is advised.

Business planning usually involves outside legal and/or consulting expertise, which requires some financial commitment. Therefore, both parties should agree that there is a firm basis for moving forward. Before moving forward with business plans, however, it may be appropriate to formalize the vision with a second letter of intent, backed up by the results of the strategic planning session. Once business planning is under way, both parties should reach agreement on as many issues as possible. However, the task force may identify certain key issues that may need to be left for future negotiation. These issues may include, for example, asset valuation and physician compensation (as discussed in chapter 4).

Both parties develop and agree to financial and operational assumptions for the collaborative entity that will drive the market and financial analysis. These assumptions include product lines, purchaser contracts, patient volumes, and service sites. Once these are established, a three- to five-year financial analysis of the collaborative relationship can be developed showing the potential impact to the parties. Because of the quantitative and scientific orientation of physicians, this approach is very appealing and conducive to furthering the discussions. Often objections and issues can be addressed by formulating multiple financial scenarios.

Financial analysis of this nature requires an assessment of the market, including volume and pricing of future business, with particular emphasis on the addition (or loss) of business due to the partnership. The real benefit of the relationship may lie several years in the future, when revenue streams under the current business structures are anticipated to be at risk.

On the expense side, planners may consolidate services or personnel functions, which will result in savings. Conversely, the plan may be to expand aggressively into new markets and services, incurring additional capital and operating expenses. Expenses should be estimated over a time frame of several years, coinciding with revenue assumptions. Capital needs and financing sources also need to be considered. For example, tax-exempt financing may be an opportunity, depending on the structure contemplated. The magnitude of capital needs will be a factor in evaluating structural options.

Ultimately, the parties may wish to compare the anticipated performance under the collaboration with performance of the respective parties without collaboration. This comparative analysis requires relatively sophisticated financial modeling, including extensive assumptions regarding both revenues and expenses. It also requires extensive knowledge of the historical performance and financial circumstances of both entities. This information is gathered as part of the due diligence that occurs concurrently with the business planning and is discussed in the next section. Information compiled from the comparative analysis is used in three ways:

1. It allows both parties to look forward and project the financial implications of working together, compared with those of maintaining the status quo.
2. This model enables the participants to carefully think through market and operational issues related to the integration.
3. It facilitates consideration of legal and organizational options in light of the strategic operational and financial priorities as specified.

Certain unresolved issues will also affect the financial picture. These include legal structures, physician compensation arrangements, practice purchases, and new program development (discussed in chapter 4). As these issues are negotiated, additional financial scenarios can be developed and reviewed by the respective parties.

Due Diligence

In terms of structuring a hospital–physician affiliation, due diligence typically consists of three components of review: business and financial issues, legal liability and compliance issues, and clinical issues. A variety of relevant information (see figure 2-3) is reviewed to determine what questions need to be anticipated with regard to a potential collaboration. On-site visits are then scheduled to gather more specific information and observe practice operations. Because of the number and diversity of potential issues, more than one visit may be required. It may be necessary to form a due diligence team made up of individuals with expertise in several different areas. For example, the first visit may entail assessment of practice operations, and the second visit may assess coding, billing, and reimbursement areas, in which case, a physician and/or utilization review nurse may be involved in a separate clinical review function. Subsequent to these visits and various follow-up calls to clarify key information, the due diligence team reports its observations and any issues that need to be raised.

An example of such an issue is the following: In the Midwest Medical Center case study (chapter 6), the initial purchases of practices presumed that the majority of all patients who had records at the existing practice would transfer to the new group practice setting. This led to exaggerated estimates of patient volume and revenues from the group practice developed through the integration of existing practices into a single practice

Figure 2-3. Sample of Practice Information Needed for Due Diligence Review

Financial

- 3–5 years financial statements/tax returns
- Depreciation schedule
- Managed care payment/bonus reports
- Leases (building and equipment)
- Insurance policies
- Scrutiny of revenues and expenses for physician net benefit
- Physician compensation and benefits; activity schedules
- Benefit plans
- Revenue breakdowns

Practice Management

- Superbill
- Policies and procedures, employee manual
- Payer mix, patient origins
- Employee information—position, compensation, benefits
- Aged trial balance report, by payer

- Procedure productivity report, by physician
- Procedure code report, with associated charges
- Organizational chart
- OSHA exposure control plan (blood-borne pathogens)
- Appropriate CLIA documentation

Clinical

- Physician credentialing information
- Audit of sample of medical charts
- Documentation of malpractice/medical legal issues

Legal/Contractual

- Leases
- Employment agreements (both practice employees and employers)
- Partnership and shareholder agreements
- Articles of incorporation
- Managed care agreements and associated schedules
- Other major contractual commitments

LIBRARY
College of St. Francis
JOLIET, ILLINOIS

156,524

site. As of this writing, Midwest Medical Center is reviewing patient records, activity levels, and transferability much more thoroughly prior to establishing forecasts for the financial impact of integrating existing practices into the group.

Due diligence, then, is an essential component of the research and planning process. Specifically, due diligence serves four purposes:

1. To improve the estimate of future business and financial performance, based on accurate knowledge of current practice operations
2. To identify practice transition and integration issues and needs
3. To identify potential risk and regulatory compliance liabilities
4. To identify clinical issues that might affect the collaboration partners

Some of these areas are explained briefly in the following subsections. Note that the due diligence review with regard to risk liability is not meant to substitute for a comprehensive legal review (described later in this chapter and in chapter 5).

Business, Financial, and Transition Issues
From a business and financial standpoint, practice production revenues and expenses can be compared with regional and national averages for the specialty. Revenue sources need to be scrutinized for transferability and future risk. This comparison and scrutiny often results in the identification of potential business and operational problems.

Billing, coding, and reimbursement are usually primary areas of interest because inappropriate coding, inadequate medical records documentation, and/or an inadequate practice fee structure can have significant impact on financial performance. Common problems include rejected claims, poor accounts receivable management, and/or the potential for missing charges. Overall practice efficiency including scheduling, computer hardware and software performance, facility layout, policies and procedures, and telephone techniques needs to be examined. In addition, personnel issues (staffing, pay levels, job functions, and the like) must be scrutinized. Pension and benefit plans can also be a major consideration in structuring the ultimate transaction.

Legal Liability and Regulatory Compliance Issues
The relevance of legal and regulatory compliance issues depends on the type of affiliation. Contractual relationships typically involve less due diligence of this nature than do asset purchases, and stock purchases require quite extensive due diligence efforts on the part of the purchaser. It is strongly recommended that each organization consult with experienced legal counsel to identify the appropriate scope of legal and contractual due diligence.

Among the common due diligence issues of this nature, other than the clinical issues identified in the next section, are safety issues as mandated by OSHA, equal opportunity and access requirements as outlined by the Americans with Disabilities Act (ADA), and the Clinical Laboratory Improvement Amendments (CLIA). Existing employee benefit plans should be reviewed for compliance with the requirements of the Employee Retirement Income Security Act (ERISA). Additionally, all parties should be required to identify past and existing lawsuits, as well as outstanding issues that had significant potential to be a lawsuit. Finally, it is extremely important that the medical practice compliance with Medicare and other payer billing rules and regulations be scrutinized. Noncompliance can result in an audit, and significant financial settlements could be required of the physician in the future.

Clinical Issues
To address common credentialing and malpractice issues, physicians generally are evaluated through the medical staff credentialing process. In addition, however, other clinical practice personnel may require a similar review process.

A medical records review is also becoming more commonplace. These reviews should be performed by experienced clinicians and/or medical auditors. In addition, it is important to analyze quality measures currently available to the practice including, for example, patient satisfaction surveys and managed care "report cards." Reviewers look for quality and appropriateness of care and levels of utilization, particularly in a managed care environment.

In summation, a good due diligence review should have four results. The first should be an evaluation of the current business and financial performance of the practice and an assessment of implications of future performance. This result relates back to the business plan for the affiliation and can be used to modify some of the financial assumptions—for example, expected patient volume or revenue—if necessary. Second, transition issues that affect the mechanics of integration (such as conversion of computer systems, personnel changes, billing systems, and so forth) should be identified. Third, any clinical and legal issues that require resolution should be identified. The fourth result, often overlooked, should be a meeting with the physician leader(s) for the purpose of communicating results of the due diligence review. It is important that this session be conducted in a clear, substantive, nonthreatening, and positive fashion.

Organizational and Legal Assessment

The organizational and legal assessment go hand in hand because of the variety of legal issues that affect individual relationship structures (detailed in chapters 3 and 5). In addition to legal issues, several other key factors drive the affiliative relationship. Some of these factors are the physician's (or group's) desire for autonomy, the hospital's desire to "lock up" the practice so the physician cannot leave or sell his or her interest, the need to control costs, the need to structure effective incentives for all parties so that the business objectives of the relationship are achieved, available capital, and reimbursement issues. (These issues and options also are discussed in chapter 3.)

Certain key negotiation issues can affect the organizational structure. The most important of these include control and decision making, ownership, physician compensation, and asset transaction and valuation. These should be omitted from this stage of the business planning process as much as possible, with the general acknowledgment that they are extremely critical and controversial issues and therefore should be negotiated in good faith by both parties only when (and if) there is mutual agreement that the overall business relationship warrants doing so.

☐ Reevaluation

Although negotiation over the key terms of the relationship has not yet taken place, it is important that the parties return to the table after the business planning process and, based on results of analysis to date, reaffirm the appropriateness of moving forward. If the collaboration involves a relatively small number of physicians (perhaps 10 to 12), this can be done informally, that is, without setting up a separate step. With a large physician group and diverse interests, however, this reevaluation phase represents a critical step in the process.

Based on the organizational options and financial analysis, the parties can now evaluate the potential relationship and the impact of specific scenarios. Although the task force has identified key issues and items to be negotiated, in some cases it makes sense to review with the entire constituency the process to date, the various options, and the rationale for the direction identified. If this is the case, the parties revisit the original objectives and evaluate whether the proposed relationship will move both parties in the right direction.

Before getting down to actual negotiation, it may be appropriate for the parties to formally indicate their interest in moving forward to the negotiation phase. In some cases, this indication of interest takes the form of a shareholder vote among physicians. In addition, the group should set (or reset) time frames for negotiation and implementation.

☐ Negotiation and Issue Resolution

At this point, both parties already should be "sold" on the vision and benefits of the proposed relationship. If this is the case, key business issues and contingency issues can be addressed.

Key Business Issues

The most complex issues—physician compensation, practice valuation, ancillary services, for example—are saved for this negotiation-and-resolution stage for three key reasons:

1. Only at this stage can mutual benefits of the relationship be understood and measured against potential trade-offs.
2. Positive momentum has been established, creating a productive environment for negotiation.
3. Task force representatives have earned credibility with their constituencies and with one another.

A fourth reason for reserving these complex issues is that, depending on the structure and desired relationship, some of these issues may not need to be negotiated. For example, certain structures may not require a practice purchase or detailed physician compensation methodologies. If potentially controversial business issues are taken on too early, they can create a divisive negotiation climate and may kill the deal.

Again, the catalysts for a healthy negotiation environment are to understand each party's needs and to look for a win–win solution. Although this may sound simple, in practice it is a very challenging assignment. Options and methods for resolving key business issues are outlined in chapter 4.

Hospital administrators must be aware that the relationship needs to be a partnership. Physicians control utilization, and thus their decisions and judgment are essential to a competitive health care system. If discussions reach a stalemate, return to the original objectives outlined at the beginning of the planning process. In the long term, there are no win–lose scenarios; they are either win–win or lose–lose for all concerned. Therefore, good faith, flexibility, and trust should prevail throughout all phases of the process.

Contingency Issues

Once key business issues are resolved, a number of adjunct "what-if" questions may be introduced by attorneys for the respective parties. These questions, distinct from the review for overall legal liability mentioned earlier, have to do with protections for the parties in the event of unexpected or undesired events—contingencies—and can be crucial should the relationship go astray. A common example is restrictive provisions on physicians should they leave the arrangement and return to practice in competition with the new relationship.

Negotiation over contingencies can sink an otherwise sound deal. Sometimes this outcome may be the only appropriate resolution because for whatever reason the parties may not be comfortable enough with one another to share fates. Ultimately these issues must be kept in perspective, for no relationship is without risk, and neither party can fully protect itself against all possible contingencies. Parties, however, can carefully assess the overall advantages of the prospective relationship against the status quo. They also can keep in mind that although circumstances may not be compelling enough to go forward with the integration at the present time, the change can be reconsidered at a later point in time.

The best way to reach final agreement is for each task force or negotiating team member to sign off on the agreed-upon terms of the business relationship by initialing the outline of the deal and later memorializing the effort into a legal document. The legal documentation step may require further analysis and negotiation, because as a rule all the "what-ifs" are incorporated into the documentation. These arrangements obviously need to be ratified by the respective constituencies, which again may require additional meetings and clarification of issues.

Throughout all steps of negotiation and resolution, the parties must remember to avoid sacrificing their future good business relationship by antagonistic or negative negotiations. The goal is to consummate the negotiation process with a hospital–physician marriage that hopefully will be the start to a new and lasting relationship.

□ Implementation

When implementing integrated relationships, there are two important considerations. One is the establishment of operational standards, and the other is transition efforts.

Establishment of Operational Standards

The establishment of operational standards for the new combined entity embraces a number of elements. Among them are standards of operation; design of financial management, billing, and information systems; managed care relationships; and personnel practices and procedures. This is much less of an issue if the hospital or health system already has an integrated practice in place that can serve as a model. If not and multiple practices are being integrated into the organization, or if a single group practice is being integrated but is short of being the "ideal practice," the organization must establish operational standards. Once standards have been set, the transition team will be more effective in evaluating the needs and integrating the practices into the larger system.

Transition

Given that the parties are still in the trust-building stage, it is important to avoid creating expectations that cannot be met. The transition phase often involves significant efforts related to conversion of computerized systems (for example, billing and accounts receivable or medical records), provider registration, new offices, personnel changes, management integration, and so on. A number of issues should be addressed, including benefit plans, salary levels, policies and procedures, managed care contracting status, and personnel benefits and policies. Transition is a difficult and traumatic undertaking for physicians and their office staff because physicians are directly and personally vested in their practices, personnel, and policies and procedures. The transition process needs to be handled delicately.

To ease the task of transition, it is helpful to discuss with physicians the complexities associated with transition during the negotiation process. If physician expectations are realistic up front, the transition can be easier for both parties.

Finally, it is extremely advantageous to have a billing system in place prior to transition. Each practice transition is unique with its inherent complications, and it is best not to implement too many practice transitions and new undertakings (for example, billing systems) at the same time. The resulting problems can be multiplicative, and attempting to do so can end the honeymoon abruptly.

□ Conclusion

The process for discussion and negotiation of a hospital–physician integration is the most essential element in achieving success. Although an attempt has been made in this chapter to outline a procedural prototype, in reality the circumstances are varied and unique to each situation. Hospital and physician group needs differ among and between one another, as do their cultural environments. The best result is built on trust, flexibility, multiple options, and compromise.

Bibliography

Benvenuto, J. A., Radoccia, R. A., and Stark, M. J. From 12 solo practices to a hospital-based LMSG in 100 easy steps. *Medical Group Management Journal* 38(4):84, 86, 88, 90, 92, July–Aug. 1991.

Cochrane, J. D. "Clinic without walls"–A futuristic model? *Integrated Healthcare Report*, Dec. 1992, pp. 1–7.

Goldstein, D. E., and McKell, D. C. *Medical Staff Alliances: How to Build Successful Partnerships with Your Physicians.* Chicago: American Hospital Publishing, 1990.

Health systems perspectives on control. *Integrated Healthcare Report*, Nov. 1992, pp. 1–5.

Herron, A. J., and Barkley, D. Forming and financing a group practice startup. *Integrated Healthcare Report*, Sept. 1992, pp. 6–10.

Herron, A. J., and Griffin, F. T., Jr. "Group without walls:" New frontier in Arizona. *Integrated Healthcare Report*, Nov. 1992, pp. 6–7.

Korenchuk, K. *Transforming the Delivery of Healthcare: Mergers, Acquisitions, and the Physician Hospital Organization.* Englewood, CO: Medical Group Management Association, 1992.

Larkin, H. Networks boost office oversight: Practices coming under more scrutiny from managed care. *American Medical News* 34:17–19, Oct. 14, 1991.

Chapter 3

Organizational Options

Factors described in chapter 1 are driving hospitals and physicians into more integrated relationships. The degree of integration is a function of complex elements that differ widely in each case. A wide range of organizational options continues to evolve, addressing these factors.

This chapter will discuss rationale for these options, beginning with a description of the levels of integration and seven major factors that influence each level. The chapter then will detail the organizational and business structures commonly used to achieve the entire spectrum of hospital–physician integration.

☐ Levels of Integration and Relationship Options

The degree of integration among hospitals and physicians ranges from loose working relationships, to codependence between and among separate entities, to full integration into a single entity. Usually the relationship begins as a loose working integration and, over time, evolves into a closer integration. Nonetheless, some current examples demonstrate movement away from full integration, often involving physicians previously employed by the hospital who are establishing separate professional corporations and contracting with their former employer hospital to provide the same services they previously offered as employees. Figure 3-1 identifies several common relationships among the three broad categories of structures and their respective levels of integration (from 0 to 10).

Working Relationship

At the lowest level of integration (0 on the scale in figure 3-1), the relationship is usually characterized as one party providing a service to the other party, with the two parties working together to achieve somewhat different goals. This level of integration and the resulting relationships are referred to as *working relationships*. A working relationship can

D. Louis Glaser of the law firm of Gardner, Carton, and Douglas, Chicago, contributed to the development of this chapter.

Figure 3-1. Levels of Integration

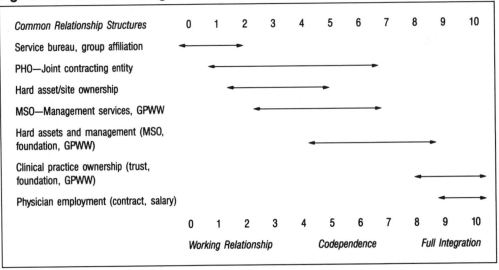

be represented by a service bureau through which a hospital provides specified services and practice enhancement to physicians.

Another form of working relationship may be the facilitation of group practice development. In this case, the hospital or health system's role is often one of education and funding outside consultants to help the physicians identify optimal group practice arrangements and strategy.

This book uses the narrow definition of *physician–hospital organization* (PHO), meaning a joint contracting entity. Under this definition, a PHO can be described as a working relationship, especially if the amount of revenue controlled through the PHO is less than 20 percent of the hospital's or physicians' revenue. As the amount of revenue derived through PHO activities increases, the relationship between physicians and the hospital becomes one of codependence.

Codependence of Separate Entities

The middle of the spectrum in figure 3-1 represents *codependence,* which is characterized by relationships between separate entities in which the parties provide needed services to each other or the services involve identical goals of the parties. For example, practice management services, offered through a management service organization (MSO) or a hospital-affiliated group practice without walls (GPWW), as well as hospital ownership of practice hard assets, represent codependent relationships. With these structures it is usually difficult—though clearly not impossible—for either party to continue without the services of the other. In fact, in markets with multiple MSOs and an unmet demand for physician services, it may be relatively easy for the physician to switch business partners.

Situations in which the hard assets of the practice are owned by the hospital, and managed by the hospital MSO, represent an even stronger integration. Furthermore, contractual relationships between the physician(s) may be long term in nature and limit a physician's ability to leave the relationship.

Stronger integration can be evidenced through ownership and control of the clinic practice by the hospital or health system. This can occur through a foundation model, a GPWW, or a trust/professional corporation, where corporate shares are held by the health system through a trust.

Full Integration

Full integration is the highest level of integration because it involves the joining of all interests within a common entity or structure. Full integration can be accomplished through physician employment, either by contract or salary, directly by the hospital. Full integration also can be achieved by a clinic or group practice's acquisition of inpatient facilities.

☐ Key Factors Influencing Levels of Integration

The degree of integration and the resulting choice of organizational structure are based on a variety of unique circumstances. Most hospital–group practice affiliations, however, are driven by the following key forces: strategic goals, physician needs, personal relationships, health care reform, marketplace and competitor activity, capital needs and resources, physician recruitment and retention, and legal issues. These factors are described in the following sections.

Strategic Goals

Larger entities, usually the hospital or health system but occasionally a physician group practice, will have identified medium- and long-term strategic goals. The strategic goals most often cited include the following:

- Increase patient volume by increasing market share or expanding into new markets.
- Develop an integrated entity to attract managed care contracts and to manage risk.
- Reduce health care delivery costs and improve efficiencies through common risk and reward incentives.

Typically, markets with greater managed care and capitation business volumes identify the second and third motivations as the primary and immediate goals, whereas less-mature managed care markets focus on the first and second strategic goals.

The strategic goals directly affect the degree of integration desired. The goal of increasing patient volume, for example, may require a less-integrated relationship. On the other hand, the motivations to attract managed care contracts and manage risk and, especially, to provide less costly and more efficient care would be best served by a stronger integration. (See figure 3-1.)

Physician Needs

Physician needs might include funding (for infrastructure or site improvements, physician recruitment, satellite site development, and so on), management expertise, payer contracting clout, and the desire to share in the savings from reduced hospital utilization under capitated contracts. Another critical physician need might be the desire for autonomy. Sometimes, physician autonomy can affect the level of integration more than any other need.

Personal Relationships

The level of rapport between the hospital and the physicians is a critical determinant of the appropriate initial relationship. The more integrated options will require greater trust, which needs to be built and nurtured over time. If a sound relationship does not already exist, less integrated options are indicated as a starting point.

Health Care Reform

Health care reform provides incentives for hospitals and physicians to form integrated delivery systems. Not only does reform implicitly favor such systems, it may provide added legal protections for certain hospital–physician activities. As of this writing, President Clinton has proposed exempting integrated health systems from state corporate practice of medicine and anti-self-referral prohibitions, thereby removing certain barriers to integration.

Market and Competitor Activity

Regardless of legislative health reform initiatives, the activities of payers and purchasers are driving change in most markets. Hospitals and physicians are evaluating their prospects for future success based on activity in the market. In many cases, fear of "being left behind" can overcome other hesitancies about the relationship. This is not always good, because many poorly conceived relationships will fail to survive the test of market forces. Nevertheless, there is some value to moving quickly and effectively. In situations with a more intense market and more competitive pressures, and/or where the parties are currently not in a market leadership position, a rapid evolution to full integration could create a competitive advantage, if successfully accomplished.

Capital Needs and Resources

Because of a variety of legal issues, less integrated relationships have more restrictions on the flow of funding. Group practices, clearly an important and competitively superior structure for health care delivery, require investment and retained earnings. Stringent legal and tax limitations, however, may inhibit investment on the part of the better capitalized hospitals in the physician entities that typically need this capital.

Because of this, hospitals often attempt to acquire and invest in the more capital-intensive aspects of the practice, such as practice assets and management services. This too has limitations, because the hospital must charge a fair market price for its management services and use of its assets. Therefore, situations that require greater capital transfer are often structured as more fully integrated relationships. Moreover, more fully integrated relationships may be able to take advantage of tax-exempt financing. This in turn provides tax-exempt hospitals with the advantage of utilizing a less expensive source of funding for capital projects.

Physician Recruitment and Retention

Competition for new physicians, especially primary care physicians, is becoming increasingly fierce. Specialists and multispecialty group practices have joined the competition for recruiting new primary care physicians who will provide a stream of referrals. Physicians who have recently completed their residencies desire salaried arrangements within a group practice. In many markets, there are few large or even medium-size group practices. Because of the capital required in starting and maintaining a group practice, greater levels of integration are often required.

Legal Issues

Legal issues affecting the choice of organizational structure are outlined in chapter 5. These issues routinely should be factored in after the business issues have been addressed. Given the ambiguity and the constantly changing nature of the law in these areas, it is exceedingly difficult to structure a relationship in a manner that entails no legal risk. The key, however, is to minimize risk through careful analysis and planning, choice of appropriate structure and contractual relationships, and clear and accurate documentation.

☐ Organizational Options

The options discussed in the following sections range from the lowest level of integration, practice enhancement services, to full integration through direct employment of physicians by the hospital or hospital ownership of physician groups. Hospital administrators throughout the country have reported a rapid increase in their desire to develop these relationships as shown in figure 3-2, which provides the results of a 1993 survey of administrators' intentions to develop these entities.

Practice Enhancement Services/Service Bureau

Often, the first substantive involvement in medical practices on the part of hospitals is through *practice enhancement services*. These services usually are provided by dedicated personnel called physician representatives, physician liaisons, or practice consultants who work with the medical staff and outside physicians to enhance their relationship with the hospital. The goal is to establish and maintain physicians' dedication and commitment to the hospital. This "physician bonding" program may address certain practice needs of the physicians, including patient referral services, educational seminars on coding and medical records documentation, practice assessments, and physician recruitment assistance. The specific services offered are often the result of a needs assessment or medical staff survey. Usually these services are offered directly by the hospital or an existing related entity, the service bureau. A separate organizational structure, created exclusively for these limited services, is rare.

Figure 3-3 is a graphic representation of the *service bureau* relationship, identifying the services most commonly offered by hospitals. In practice, hospitals often charge a minimal amount or sometimes nothing for some enhancement services, often because they are broadly applied and available to the medical staff as a whole. Legal restrictions, however, dictate that the physician(s) must pay fair market value for receipt of practice enhancement services. For example, where consulting services are engaged for the exclusive benefit of a specific physician, he or she should be charged all of the costs incurred.

Figure 3-2. Hospital Intentions to Develop Hospital–Physician Organizations

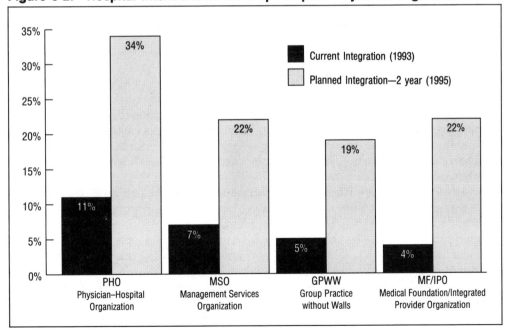

Note: This survey is based on 507 CEO responses.

Source: Report on hospital–physician integration survey. *CPA Health Niche Advisor* 10: 1, 4, 1993.

Figure 3-3. Practice Enhancement Services Offered by a Service Bureau

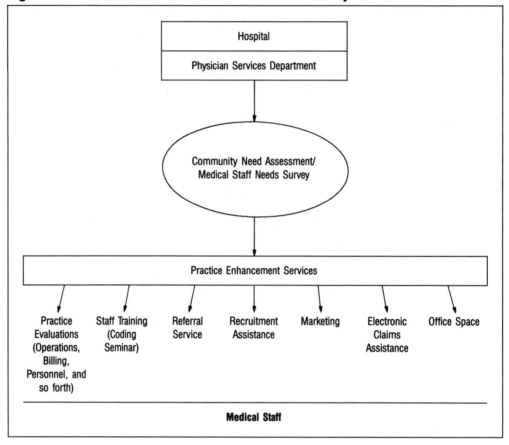

The service bureau is a tactical step in the direction of improved integrated relationships and in time may lead to wider integration. Executed properly, the service bureau accomplishes a number of important goals, such as building trust and providing physician assistance as needed. However, the service bureau also has significant limitations as listed in figure 3-4.

PHO, a Joint Contracting Entity

A *PHO* is a legal entity (corporation, partnership, limited liability corporation, or unincorporated association) formed between a hospital and physician group to achieve shared market objectives and other mutual interests. Ownership and control usually are shared 50/50 between the physicians and hospital, although it is not uncommon for the hospital to own up to 80 percent. Most often the physicians, composed largely of the hospital's medical staff, maintain independence and ownership of their group practice. Physician members agree to have the PHO negotiate managed care contracts within certain prespecified parameters.

Areas around the country that do not yet have significant group practice development and managed care penetration are "bingeing" on PHO development. These areas, which typically have had less hospital–physician integration and a preponderance of solo practices, are carefully testing the integration waters by creating this separate entity for the purpose of negotiating managed care contracts.

The value of the PHO structure is currently the focal point of debate, much of which centers on dissatisfaction with the PHO as a viable, long-term entity within a managed care system. The criticism is valid because of the entity's inherent weaknesses—lack of integration and lack of real improvement to the cost structure of health care delivery, to name two. However, in many less developed managed care markets, the PHO structure

Figure 3-4. Capabilities and Limitations of the Service Bureau Model

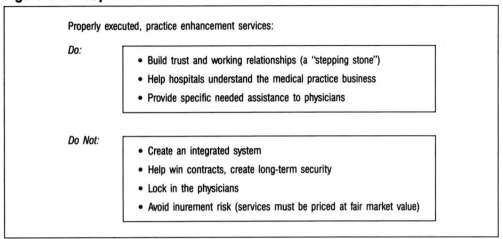

Properly executed, practice enhancement services:

Do:
- Build trust and working relationships (a "stepping stone")
- Help hospitals understand the medical practice business
- Provide specific needed assistance to physicians

Do Not:
- Create an integrated system
- Help win contracts, create long-term security
- Lock in the physicians
- Avoid inurement risk (services must be priced at fair market value)

is an excellent transitional vehicle for organizational change. At a minimum, it is both an educational forum and a forum for initiating cooperation between physicians and hospitals. In this fashion, the PHO functions as a conduit to reposition health care providers into more integrated structures. In addition, the more successful PHOs establish participation criteria that promote cost-effective care, contract with purchasers, evaluate individual and collective performance, and effect the resultant financial distribution. Some parameters for PHO development are described in the following sections.

Process and Timing
Typically the PHO development process represents the hospital's and physicians' first comprehensive effort at integration. Therefore, a significant mutual education and goal-setting effort is required initially. In addition, a coordinated managed care strategy should be developed, one based on research of market conditions. This enables the planning group to review alternative structures for the PHO as outlined later in this section.

Once the appropriate structure is selected, a business plan for PHO operations needs to be established that incorporates criteria for physician participation, negotiation ranges for fees, and identification of a budget for capitalization and operation. The business plan also serves as important documentation that the arrangement is being structured in compliance with legal requirements. In particular, the business plan should demonstrate that capitalization and operation of the PHO does not result in the physicians receiving impermissible benefits in violation of fraud and abuse laws or in a manner that could jeopardize the hospital's tax-exempt status.

In terms of timing, PHO planning and development is a three-to-five-month process, depending on the size of the task force, its familiarity with the issues, and participant motivations. Implementation can take an additional two to four months, depending on information systems requirements.

PHO Functions
The function of the PHO is to act as a "front organization" or manager for managed care contracting and administration. The key to success involves the organization's ability to market itself and to profitably manage the care of the defined population; that is, the population assigned by the purchaser. To do this, the PHO has the following responsibilities:

- *Internal financial arrangements:* Initially, the PHO establishes a range of fees acceptable to physicians, hospital(s), and other health care providers. Once the minimum acceptable fee is established, the PHO can negotiate contracts in conformance with these guidelines. Other key contract terms such as withholdings, risk and bonus arrangements, reinsurance, stop-loss protection, and "nonrisk" services are negotiated accordingly.

- *Utilization review:* The PHO establishes credentialing standards and collects utilization data, as well as cost and quality information from the contracted providers, and in closed panel (selective) PHOs, recredentials physicians according to predetermined performance criteria. In some cases, incentive payments are based on performance criteria, although this is more common in more fully integrated relationships.
- *Billing and disbursement:* The PHO bills the payers, manages financial assets, and disburses funds to contracted providers according to preagreed terms.
- *Marketing:* The PHO markets its provider panel services to payers, focusing on the provider quality and cost-effectiveness.
- *Contract review and negotiation:* PHO personnel review both business and legal terms of contracts with purchasers, sometimes requiring outside assistance.
- *Planning:* The PHO functions as a focal point for medium- and long-term collaborative planning between the hospital and physicians.

Cost and Capitalization
The financial needs of the PHO vary, depending (among other factors) on the volume of managed care contracts and business available through the PHO. Typically, $100,000 to $300,000 is enough to set up the PHO, develop the contracts, and implement systems. Operating expenses also vary and usually will be funded by a percentage of revenues (typically 2 to 8 percent). If this business is capitated, operating expenses are immediately funded. Other managed care contracts will require additional working capital in the PHO.

Depending on the volume and nature of the contracts, the PHO can contract with outside vendors, including third-party payers, to handle its information system requirements. The more capitation and/or global contracts, the greater the financial incentive to bring the services in-house in order to maximize profits.

The necessary funds can be advanced through a loan from the hospital or direct capitalization. The hospital's share of capitalization usually ranges from 50 to 80 percent. Conversely, the physicians contribute from 20 to 50 percent of the capital. The lower physician contribution of 20 percent is typical when PHO ownership is limited to a smaller number of primary care physicians. Although some PHOs require no physician contributions, a typical capital contribution toward a PHO appears to be between $300 and $1,000 per physician; occasionally it is higher.

Critical to the capitalization of a PHO in which physicians are to have an ownership interest is that the hospital's risk (that is, capital contributed) must be in proportion to its return (ownership interest and right to distributions). The physician-owners also must truly be "at risk" for their investment. In essence, the hospital must examine its investment in the PHO as it would any other investment in a for-profit enterprise. In the absence of the required protections, the structure is likely to create significant legal risk for participants. If money is loaned by the hospital as initial capital, the loan must be at a market interest rate and contain commercially reasonable terms. If not, the hospital faces similar legal risks.

Initial and continuing costs of a PHO are often offset through use of hospital personnel. For example, a portion of a hospital employee's salary may be paid by the PHO, which enables the PHO to benefit from the involvement of skilled professionals without incurring costs associated with hiring full-time employees. If this is done, however, the PHO is obligated to enter into an employee leasing agreement with the hospital that provides for adequate reimbursement of hospital employee expenses. Otherwise, the arrangement may be subject to tax and fraud and abuse problems.

Participation in the PHO
The two options for membership in a PHO are open panels, which allow every member of the medical staff access, and closed panels, which restrict physician participation based

on preestablished criteria. The differences between these panels are explained in the following sections.

Open Panel

A typical PHO structure is identified in figure 3-5. In most markets the fastest, easiest way to develop the PHO is to allow all medical staff members to participate in the panel, thus creating an *open-panel PHO*. Usually this involves minimal credentialing, as defined in figure 3-6. Criteria for participation frequently are the same used for medical staff membership.

A variation of the open-model PHO is the imposition of credentialing over time. As data are accumulated on the providers, a comparative database can be established, with standards set against which participants are measured. In reality, these standards are difficult to set after formation of the PHO. In addition, physician removal from the PHO can be a difficult process that involves a legal proceeding, particularly if the impact on that physician's business is significant or results in his or her removal from the medical staff.

A third option in an open-panel PHO is to create credentialed subpanels. In essence, the PHO identifies additional, more restrictive criteria and evaluates its membership against these criteria. A subset of the PHO physicians is identified that meets these criteria, and that subpanel participates in the plan or contract. This enables groups of PHO members to be aggregated based on more restrictive criteria over time, and the PHO can market

Figure 3-5. Typical Physician–Hospital Organization (PHO) Structure

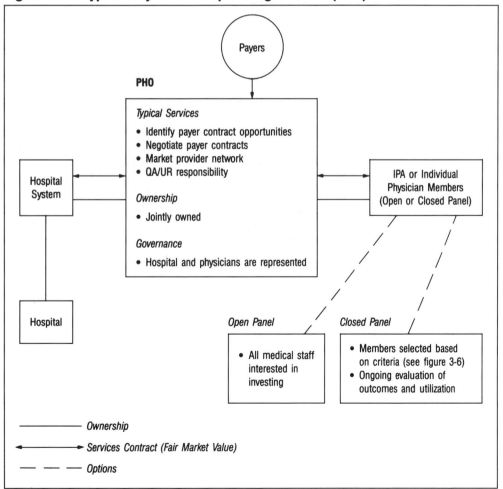

Figure 3-6. PHO Physician Credentialing Criteria

Minimal Criteria

Open Panel

1. Valid and current medical and DEA license
2. Must have no history of convictions by state or federal agency for fraud, inurement, or criminal activity
3. No significant history of sanctions, disciplinary actions, suspensions, or revocations by hospital, HMO, state licensing boards, peer review committee, or insurance companies
4. Satisfactory review of malpractice claims
5. Minimum professional liability requirement (that is, $1 million per occurrence and $3 million aggregate)

Restrictive PHOs

6. Open to "active-status" medical staff only
7. Adhere to more stringent utilization review and quality assurance guidelines established by the PHO
8. Board certification required
9. Specific physician specialty(s) only (for example, primary care)
10. Individual physician performance standards based on charges per case, intensity of ancillary utilization, LOS, and/or mortality

Closed Panel

11. Direct chart analysis and peer evaluation
12. Patient and consumer satisfaction survey results
13. Outcome studies and compliance with case maps

Most Stringent

different provider combinations. On the downside, this is a complicated management undertaking and does not enable the PHO to have a clear and positive identity with payers and purchasers.

Overall, open-panel PHOs tend to attract a lot of specialists and high utilizers. The high-quality, cost-efficient physicians may also be a part of the PHO but will have other attractive options. Over time, the primary care physicians understand that they are at risk based on the overall performance of the PHO and will seek more selective and cost-effective quality panels. As a result, open-panel PHOs lose the most desirable physicians and, thus, lose their competitive appeal.

In an open PHO, physicians are sometimes represented by an independent physician association or physician organization (IPA or PO), under which the hospital shares control and decision making equally. Creation of such an entity, representing the constituent physicians, often creates a hierarchy that can make PHO development discussions (and management) much easier. In other cases, however, the IPA can be an additional layer of bureaucracy, resulting in an adversarial environment that contributes to costly delays to PHO decision making. Here again there is no "right" approach—the organizational approach needs to fit the circumstances.

Closed Panel

Limited-participation PHOs, or *closed-panel PHOs*, can be based on different criteria—less stringent criteria (board certification or board eligibility) or more stringent criteria (economic credentialing criteria, length of stay, cost per case, clinical protocol adherence, and so forth). Figure 3-6 identifies some criteria used to credential physicians selectively.

The task of the closed-panel PHO is to credential physicians up front and screen out low-quality or high-cost physicians. The problem is that the PHO often does not have good data for this screening at the outset. Some utilization data, however, are available through hospital information systems, and even better data are controlled by major payers, although not often made available unless the payer is a party to the relationship.

Another increasingly popular option in the closed-panel PHO is to limit specialty membership. This enables the PHO to develop a provider panel that makes it attractive to the payers. For example, one option is to limit physician participation in PHOs to primary care physicians and OB/GYN physicians only. This structure appeals strongly to managed care payers who seek gatekeeper panels and a primary care focus.

Limiting provider participation may raise antitrust considerations, particularly if competing physicians make participation decisions about other competitors or if the PHO obtains a certain market share or concentration for a physician specialty. Accordingly, the criteria for admission and removal, as well as other relevant market information, must be analyzed for antitrust compliance.

An alternative strategy (combining both the open and closed models) is for the PHO to measure physicians against key credentialing criteria up front, giving all interested physicians an opportunity to understand and improve against these criteria. After one year of contingent membership in the PHO, physicians are evaluated based on the previous year's activities. If the physician measures up, he or she becomes a full member of the PHO. This enables the physicians to be educated on the factors important to the PHO and to modify their behavior within a defined time frame to meet the criteria and become part of the PHO.

Other Issues

Certain other issues are relevant to PHO integration. These include control, legal mandates, and business volumes, as discussed in the following list:

- *Control:* The failure of many previously established IPA models was the dominance of specialty physicians. Primary care physicians should have strong, if not dominant, input in the PHO. Although the PHO represents shared hospital and physician control, a common problem is that physicians cannot agree on who among them will participate on a PHO board of directors. In such a case, the board size can be expanded to accommodate more physician participation. Nonetheless, their collective vote would still amount to only 50 percent (or perhaps their percentage of capital contributed), thus maintaining the parity between physician and hospital control, but enabling more physicians to participate at the board level. As board size increases, however, the efficiency with which it operates will diminish significantly.
- *Legal mandates:* As detailed in chapter 5, antitrust issues often emerge in PHO discussions. In addition, some states require the PHO to be licensed as an HMO to accept capitated contracts. In these cases, the PHO is burdened with licensure requirements, typically requiring the availability of significant funding reserves. Finally, federal income tax and fraud and abuse concerns are present in PHOs involving physician ownership.
- *Business volumes:* To maintain the interest and involvement of constituent physicians, the PHO needs to direct enough business to have an impact on the participants. A properly structured PHO should be an outgrowth of a managed care strategy and be competitive and successful in gaining significant contracts within one year of implementation. However, expectations need to be managed so that the effort is not considered a failure if the first year does not result in desired contract volumes. Many PHOs do not garner significant business until the second year and beyond.

Summary of PHO Model

As identified in figure 3-7, PHOs accomplish a limited set of goals. They do not achieve a fully integrated system and, when poorly executed, they can inhibit an organization's

Figure 3-7. Capabilities and Limitations of the PHO Model

Properly executed, the PHO:

Does:

- Develop collaboration and trust between physician and hospital
- Improve understanding of patient management
- Provide basis for further integration
- Exclude (or improve) poor performers
- Attract managed care contracts

Does Not:

- Enable major investment in physician practice
- Integrate the physicians' and hospital's interest
- Significantly control/change practice patterns
- Reduce costs/consolidate services

ability to compete in the future health care environment and negatively affect collaborative relationships with the physician participants. In less mature markets PHOs are effective and well recommended, with the caveat that *there must be selectivity* in the physician panels sooner rather than later. Also, PHOs should be seen as a stepping-stone to more fully integrated relationships in the future.

Hospital Ownership of Practice Site and Assets

A further step toward integration involves *hospital ownership of medical practice sites and hard assets,* with the physician leasing practice assets from the hospital. Accordingly, the physician remains in full control of, as well as retains ownership of, other aspects of the practice; employs the staff; and directly bills the payers. This situation typically arises out of one of two circumstances. Either a retiring physician sells his or her hard assets and building to the hospital and the hospital identifies an existing physician or new recruit to work in the practice, or a new hospital-developed site is established and a physician works in the practice, sometimes on a part-time "time-share" basis.

Although this is often seen as a temporary arrangement on the part of the hospital, it is increasingly a permanent arrangement, especially in semirural and rural areas. Figure 3-8 depicts the typical arrangement under this structure.

Costs to the hospital are the capital cost of purchasing the hard assets, the lease cost of the building or office space, building maintenance and utility costs, and leasehold improvements if any. From a legal standpoint, the hospital must charge fair market value for use of the space and assets. In practice, however, significant variation is seen in the costs charged to the physician. The hospital usually has a very limited supply of "willing buyers" to use the space and, if the space is used only on a part-time basis, the hospital cannot expect to recoup costs based on full-time utilization. Therefore, the hospital must document that the amounts charged, including any rental incentives, are commercially reasonable and are in line with market rates.

Although this strategy accomplishes a number of important goals, such as market penetration or practice retention (see figure 3-9), certain key features of integration are not available, such as cost reduction and alignment of hospital and physician incentives. Overall, this strategy only achieves limited tactical objectives and does not represent a secure relationship in competitive markets. Nonetheless, it may serve temporary and tactical purposes in competitive markets and be a viable long-term relationship in rural settings.

Figure 3-8.   Typical Hospital Ownership of Practice Site and Assets Structure

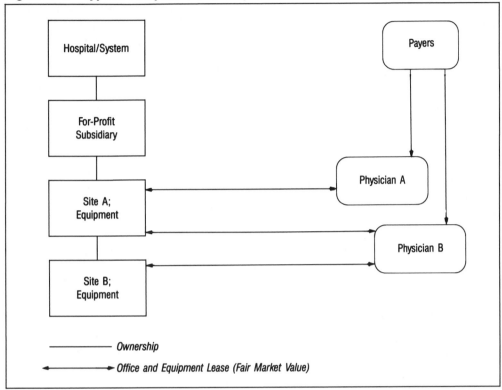

Figure 3-9.   Capabilities and Limitations of the Hospital Ownership of Practice Site and Assets Model

Properly executed, site and asset ownership:

Does:
- Allow hospital name identification and new market penetration
- Lower capital requirements of the physician

Does Not:
- Control costs or practice patterns
- Integrate the physician into a group practice arrangement
- Attract new contracts (perhaps indirectly through enhanced geographic coverage)
- Build hospital expertise in practice management

MSO Model

Management service organizations (MSOs) encompass a broad range of relationships that generally have two features in common. One, the physician or physician group has ceded day-to-day management responsibilities for the practice to the hospital or health system entity. Two, the physician or group maintains ownership of the clinical practice and bills payers directly under the physician or physician group provider number.

The MSO represents a significant step beyond practice-enhancement services. A comprehensive practice management capability is established, enabling the hospital to take over operational and financial aspects of the practice, including billing, collections, personnel, high-level management, and so forth. Physicians maintain their practice autonomy.

43

They bill the payer for services and pay the MSO a management fee (priced at fair market value). The hospital sometimes takes the risk of managing the practice for an agreed-on percentage of collections, but physicians continue to own their goodwill and patient records. A significant drawback is that the physician can walk away from this arrangement at any time.

Hospitals typically enter into an MSO relationship for any number of reasons. Among them are a desire to increase the physician's loyalty to and dependence on the hospital, to create the foundation for group practice development, to make practice management more cost-efficient, to encourage group development or expansion through use of hospital capital, to enhance physician recruitment efforts, and to create a management vehicle to conduct PHO operations.

A more fully integrated MSO relationship involves the hospital's purchase of hard assets and continued hospital capital investment in the practice assets. The greater the degree of control, the more closely the relationship begins to resemble the foundation model discussed later in this chapter.

Overall, physicians find MSOs attractive for various reasons, including improved management capabilities and personnel, high-level management, future growth potential, immediate cash payout for hard assets and/or accounts receivable, and the development of a relationship that can help them survive and thrive under health care reform.

Structure and Strategy

An MSO can be structured as a division of the hospital, a freestanding subsidiary, or a joint venture with physicians. Figure 3-10 depicts a typical MSO organizational structure. Regardless of the structure, physician representation on the board is a must, often approaching 50 percent of board representation.

Figure 3-10. Typical Management Services Organization (MSO) Structure

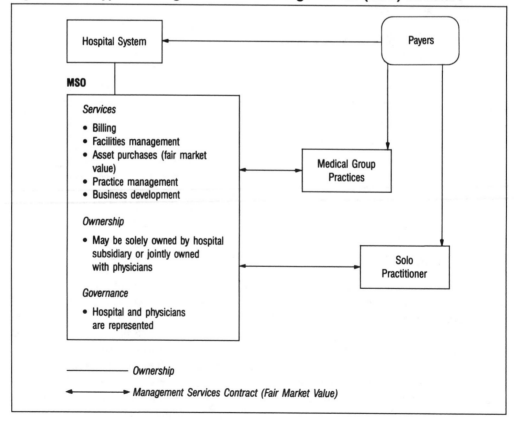

The strategy applied for physician involvement in the MSO is important. The broadest (and most difficult to manage) strategy involves management services and asset acquisition offered to any willing physician. A common variation is to limit the service to any and all primary care physicians, with no condition for further integration.

The second strategy is to offer the MSO services to physicians interested in a group practice without walls (GPWW). In this situation the hospital manages the practices of various physicians interested in integrating into a single practice. The MSO introduces common management practices and systems to the practices as a step toward integration. Over time, the physicians agree to come together as a group practice, perhaps into a single professional corporation. This intention is often identified as a precondition for physician involvement.

The third approach uses the MSO to facilitate practice site integration, as well as group practice integration. The MSO invests in carefully planned sites, and the physicians' practices are integrated into these sites and, over time, into a single group practice structure.

The second and third strategies are often called *conditional MSOs* and involve the physician in a progression toward greater integration over time. Sometimes the physician has the option to participate in the MSO for up to two years before committing to join the professional corporation and can buy back practice assets at preagreed terms if he or she chooses to opt out of the arrangement.

Another common use of the MSO is as a planned temporary developmental step toward a foundation model or full employment relationship. Because of the legal and tax issues surrounding foundation models, as well as the physicians' perceived loss of autonomy, there may be significant time delay and uncertainty regarding final approval. The MSO structure is often used to implement the relationship and integrate the practices while obtaining physician approval and/or seeking final approvals from the government.

Over time, to increase the degree of integration, the hospital may establish a hospital-affiliated professional corporation managed by the MSO. The structure through which this can be accomplished depends on state law corporate practice of medicine principles. This structure provides the hospital with greater flexibility in dealing with such issues as capital investment, compensation and cost-effectiveness issues, and other elements critical to success in a managed care environment. Physicians not included in the affiliated professional corporation can continue to take advantage of the management capabilities and sophistication of the MSO through their services contract.

Functions

The functions of the MSO are shown in figure 3-11. The MSO must engage professional management expertise capable of handling large-scale practices. Generally speaking, hospital administrators and managers of small practices are not equipped for this undertaking. It is also crucial to maintain a service orientation toward the client, that is, the physician. It is important that the first practices under the MSO management be successful because other physicians' willingness to work with the health system will be influenced by the results. Due to unavoidable obstacles typical in new business start-ups,

Figure 3-11. MSO Functions

• Practice operations	• Marketing
• Personnel	• Managed care contract negotiation (in some cases)
• Purchasing	• Asset purchase *(optional)*
• Billing/medical claims submission	• Facility management
• Collection of receivables	• Accounting
• Recruitment assistance	• Information systems

however, it is important to manage the physicians' expectations so they are realistic from the outset.

The challenge facing the MSO from the beginning is to competently manage existing practices under contract while executing the enormous task of new practice transition. This often proves to be an overwhelming task and requires qualified and adequate staffing support.

Cost and Capitalization

The cost of establishing an MSO is highly variable, as is the cost of its operation. The most influential variable is the number of physician practices under management. The scope of MSO services can range from two or three to hundreds of physicians.

A successful MSO will result in strong demand on the part of the physicians. Because of working capital requirements, rapid growth will necessitate continued losses; however, the asset value of the business, including accounts receivable and hard assets, will be growing at the same time. If physicians invest in the MSO, the hospital must ensure that its capitalization of the entity satisfies the legal requirements (where applicable) for a tax-exempt entity participating in a for-profit venture. In particular, the hospital must structure and capitalize the entity so that its risk is proportionate to its return and the physician investors are truly at risk for their investment. The hospital also must ensure that the MSO does not operate as a conduit, whereby hospital funds are continuously funneled into the MSO for subsidizing practice operations. The development of a bona fide business plan will assist in providing documentation to avoid this pitfall. If the MSO purchases practice assets, independent appraisals should be obtained to provide further documentation of the arm's-length nature of the MSO's activities.

If the hospital provides MSO services through a division or a wholly owned entity, it must ensure that the services offered by the MSO are priced at fair market value in order to avoid tax fraud and abuse. The MSO cannot function as a subsidy for the physicians purchasing services. For physicians who invest in the MSO entity, these concerns may be diminished through their participation in decision making. Nonetheless, to the extent that physician owners receive services from the MSO, the same issues will arise.

Developing a business plan, as discussed in chapters 2 and 4, will also enable potential physician investors to make informed decisions about investing in an MSO. The business plan should indicate the period of time over which the MSO will generate a return to its investors. Without such a plan, the hospital risks strained physician relations in the event the MSO fails to generate a return in the time anticipated by the physicians without benefit of the business plan.

Other Issues

An MSO can facilitate recruitment of new physicians. Newcomers to an existing practice that participates in the MSO should be faced with a much-reduced buy-in requirement because the practice no longer owns or needs to invest in hard assets. The requirement should be significantly lower than that for comparable freestanding practices.

Ultimate control of the MSO is usually maintained by the hospital, though physician input on decision making and policy remains vital. Physicians control income distribution within the group practice, although the financial incentives may or may not be consistent with managed care motivations. The MSO has only indirect influence over these issues by virtue of the practice manager's rapport and involvement with the physicians on these issues.

Summary of MSO Model

Figure 3-12 summarizes the capabilities and limitations of an MSO in hospital–group practice integration. The primary immediate benefit is improved financial performance of poorly managed solo practices and, secondarily, enhanced economies of scale through consolidation.

Figure 3-12. Capabilities and Limitations of the MSO Model

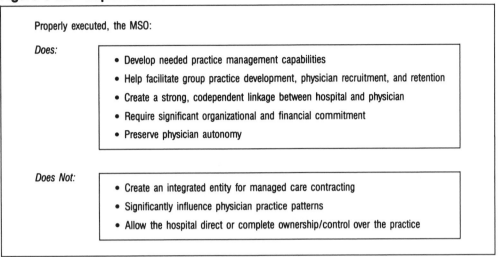

Properly executed, the MSO:

Does:
- Develop needed practice management capabilities
- Help facilitate group practice development, physician recruitment, and retention
- Create a strong, codependent linkage between hospital and physician
- Require significant organizational and financial commitment
- Preserve physician autonomy

Does Not:
- Create an integrated entity for managed care contracting
- Significantly influence physician practice patterns
- Allow the hospital direct or complete ownership/control over the practice

Achieving these goals, however, requires significant cultural adjustment on the part of physicians who have run their own practices for a long time. For example, physicians continue to want to control MSO office staff, although they no longer are their employees. This emotional reality must be understood and dealt with diplomatically.

A second problem with the MSO is that, ultimately, multiple-contracted physician groups, the hospital, and the MSO all have different leadership structures. This creates a complicated and potentially conflicting relationship among the various entities. The conflict most often relates to the percentage of revenues paid for management services, capital investment budgets, and managed care contract volume and services. In highly competitive markets, this time-consuming and unwieldy structure may prove to be a disadvantage if the competition is aligned in more efficiently integrated relationships.

Foundation Model

In the *foundation model*, medical practices are acquired and managed through a separate and (typically) not-for-profit corporation of the health system—the foundation. The foundation includes all the operational and service functions of the MSO model, plus the following added features:

- It may purchase the *entire* medical practice, including intangibles.
- It bills the payer directly for physician services.
- It may be able to benefit from tax-exempt financing.
- It may avoid corporate practice of medicine issues.

In this model, the hospital or health system benefits from the strength of the physician linkage, the ability to invest heavily in practice expansion and development while minimizing legal issues, and the ability to purchase practice intangibles (for example, goodwill) without facing corporate practice of medicine issues as discussed in chapter 5. From the physicians' perspective, they are able to realize financial gain for the entire value of the practice, continue practicing within a larger entity yet avoid direct employment by the hospital, and maintain control over income distribution among physicians.

Structure and Strategy

A typical structure for a foundation relationship is depicted in figure 3-13. The hospital or health system creates a new entity, with either the hospital or the system's parent corporation as the sole member or shareholder. The foundation may be either a for-profit

Figure 3-13. Typical Foundation Model Structure

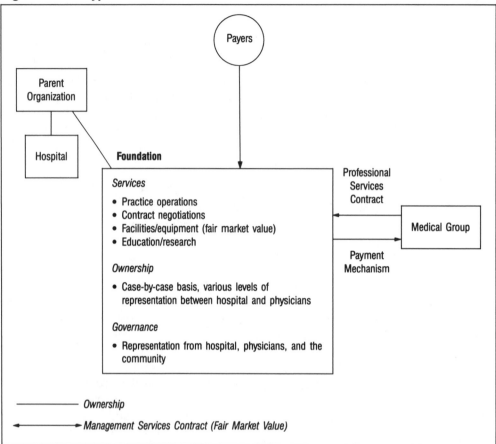

or a not-for-profit corporation, entering into a purchase agreement with an existing group practice to acquire the practice's assets. Following acquisition, the foundation enters into a contract with the group practice to provide services within the foundation's newly acquired clinics.

Perhaps the most significant advantage of creating a not-for-profit corporation is obtaining tax-exempt status and utilizing the proceeds from tax-exempt bonds to acquire the medical group assets. Tax-exempt status, however, imposes significant structural and operational limitations on the foundation. (See figure 3-14.) In particular, the foundation board is limited to 20 percent physician representation so as to comply with a standard the IRS seeks to establish as a "safe harbor." Typically the hospital or health system provides 20 percent representation, with the remaining 60 percent being unaffiliated community representatives. (This 60–40 test is discussed in chapter 5.) Physician participation in compensation decisions and on committees is prohibited.

The foundation serves as the operational, management, and payer-contracting entity of the practice. In fact, for all practical purposes, the foundation is the practice. The major exception is that physicians retain their professional corporation, which has an exclusive contract to provide medical services to the foundation. Physicians control income distribution within the professional corporation, but the level of compensation paid to the corporation is controlled by the board or a foundation committee.

Establishing a foundation model is a complicated legal undertaking. An IRS ruling may be obtained to establish the foundation's tax-exempt status, a process that has been known to take up to two years and involve significant negotiation with the IRS. The ruling, however, will not address the issue of whether amounts paid were in fact at fair

Figure 3-14. Foundation Model: Key IRS Criteria for Tax-Exempt Status

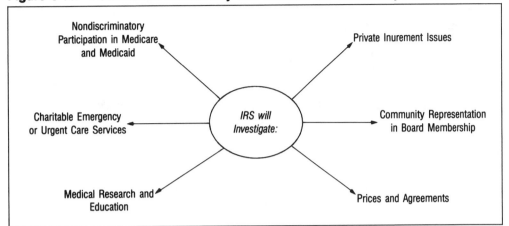

market value; this issue is left for the audit context. Moreover, the determination letter will stipulate that the favorable determination is conditioned on the transaction not violating tax fraud and abuse laws. Therefore, the value of the ruling is limited. Again, "fair market value" transactions must be documented through arm's-length negotiations, independent valuations, and market comparisons.

Practice valuation is a critical issue. Both the IRS and the Inspector General have made reference to the mechanisms of practice valuation, especially the valuation of intangible assets, and their views are not entirely consistent. To be safe, however, most foundations attempt to establish evidence that practice purchases have been at or below fair market value. Details on fair market valuation methodologies and requirements are identified in chapter 4.

In states with strong corporate practice of medicine prohibitions, the foundation is seen as a very desirable alternative. For example, in California foundation models are commonplace, both because of the market pressures for more highly integrated structures to address capitation and due to the state's having one of the strictest corporate practice of medicine laws in the country.

Cost and Capitalization
Because the foundation model may involve the purchase of tangible and intangible physician practice assets, it is a high-cost option. A major advantage of tax-exempt foundations is the availability of funding through tax-exempt bonds. This strategy has been successfully implemented in several of the California foundations.

Physician Compensation
Three common mechanisms for compensation of the physician group affiliated with the foundation model are percentage of collections; fixed fee, based on historical production and compensation levels of the physicians; and capitation payment. A combination of these methodologies may also be used. In all cases, the payment mechanism and amounts must be consistent with fair market value compensation for physicians. In integrated delivery models, and particularly under capitation, extreme ranges of physician compensation are eliminated. Therefore, industry averages and a "reasonable range" of compensation based on these averages are more acceptable guidelines.

The fact that the group controls individual physician compensation can be an advantage and a disadvantage to the affiliated lay entity. Physician compensation is one of the most controversial areas within a group practice and can cause much conflict and disharmony within a group. Leaving compensation battles to be resolved by physicians has significant advantages, especially in a newly integrated relationship.

The disadvantage, however, is that by virtue of their numbers, specialists can dominate the group. This situation may result in noncompetitive compensation for primary care physicians, thus weakening the group. A second and perhaps more dangerous risk is that physician compensation structures within the group may create incentives contrary to the foundation's goals. For example, physician payment systems may be based on the volume of services, whereas lower utilization and fewer services means greater profitability under capitation. The greatest potential weakness of the foundation model is this lack of control over individual physician compensation and the resulting organizational weaknesses.

Other Issues
Other issues to be considered include payment for lost physician ancillary revenues, long-term management of additional group integration, and physician defection. These topics are addressed in the following subsections.

Ancillary Revenues
In structuring a foundation model, a major negotiation point between a health system and physicians is payment for lost ancillary revenues. This is particularly important in larger group practices where ancillary revenues are significant. Three options are available: (1) to calculate a value for these services and include that value in the purchase price of the practice(s); (2) to provide for ongoing payment to physicians that includes an amount for ancillary services, based on pre-integration income and compensation levels; or (3) to allow the parties to combine these options. Whichever alternative is selected, the parties must address the payments in light of applicable federal and state prohibitions on physician self-referrals, such as the 1989 Ethics in Patient Referrals Act (the Stark Bill). Ancillary revenue is addressed in greater detail in chapter 4.

Long-Term Integration Management
An issue currently encountered by the early foundation models is how to handle the integration of additional groups. Management options include developing a separate foundation for other relationships, contracting with multiple groups through a single foundation, or merging all practices into a single foundation with physicians operating in one contracted professional corporation. Although the latter option is the simplest and most manageable, other more complicated relationship combinations are being implemented for various political and business reasons. The viability of these structures remains to be seen.

Physician Defection
A weakness of the foundation model is that, even though the entire practice assets have been purchased and merged into the foundation, the physician(s) may be free to leave the relationship and compete with the foundation. All parties having an interest in the foundation's long-term success must be knowledgeable about various state judicial decisions on the enforceability of noncompete covenants. In addition, within the context of tax-exempt foundation status, the IRS has questioned the permissibility of these covenants on the basis of whether they provide community benefit. As is the case generally among organizations, no integrated relationship can ensure against the defection of key participants. The difference here, however, is that the physician participants remain organized in a separate entity—the professional corporation—and could organize or threaten defection en masse.

Summary of Foundation Model
Figure 3-15 outlines the key roles of a foundation model. Overall, it has been demonstrated to be an effective vehicle for hospital–physician integration and, despite associated legal complexities, it exhibits significant added benefits, particularly tax-exempt financing.

Figure 3-15. Capabilities and Limitations of the Foundation Model

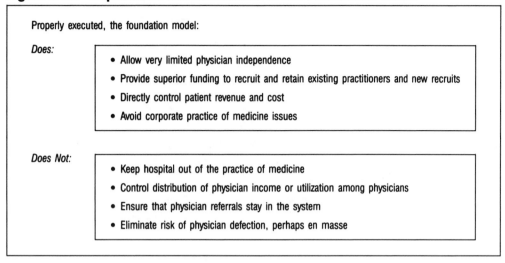

Properly executed, the foundation model:

Does:
- Allow very limited physician independence
- Provide superior funding to recruit and retain existing practitioners and new recruits
- Directly control patient revenue and cost
- Avoid corporate practice of medicine issues

Does Not:
- Keep hospital out of the practice of medicine
- Control distribution of physician income or utilization among physicians
- Ensure that physician referrals stay in the system
- Eliminate risk of physician defection, perhaps en masse

On the other hand, the model exhibits some weaknesses relative to controlling physician behavior and effective management of health care delivery.

Trust/Professional Corporation Model

The *trust/professional corporation model* enables the economic integration of hospitals and physicians in states with strong corporate practice of medicine laws. The professional corporation, under the direct control of the hospital or health system, can use the trust as a vehicle for acquiring and managing all aspects of medical practice. The adaptability of this model is dependent on state law.

Structure and Strategy
As described in figure 3-16, the hospital establishes a trust to which the hospital is the beneficiary, and a physician or physician group is designated to act as trustee. The trustee serves at the hospital's discretion and may be replaced by the hospital at any time for any reason. The trust creates a professional corporation with the physician trustee as the sole or majority shareholder on behalf of the trust. Through the trustee, the trust purchases shares in the corporation and/or makes loans to it that are sufficient for capitalization. Other physicians may also be involved and exchange the equity in their practice for corporate shares. This variation is known as the *shared equity model.*

Corporate shareholders elect the board of directors, which in turn appoints corporate officers. In some cases, depending on state law, officers and directors may be nonphysicians from the hospital's management team or board of directors.

The professional corporation then owns and operates the group practice, employs physicians, and directly contracts and bills for all professional services. Profits from practice operations, after payment of all expenses including physician compensation, can be distributed back to the shareholders (the trust included) in the form of dividends. The trust can then distribute profits back to the hospital as distribution of trust income to the beneficiary.

Function
The function of the trust/professional corporation is to own and manage medical practices. This includes all management and clinical functions, personnel, supplies, employment of physicians, and, in many cases, purchase and integration of existing practices.

Figure 3-16. Typical Trust/Professional Corporation Model Structure

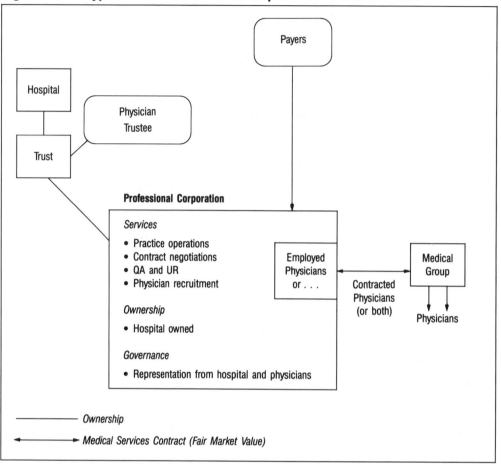

Cost and Capitalization
Because the trust/professional corporation typically either purchases tangible and intangible assets of existing practices or starts new practices, this approach requires significant capital. This capital can be in the form of a loan or direct capitalization from the shareholder(s). The costs of the trust vary, mainly depending on the following conditions:

- The existence of practice management capabilities, resources, or an MSO
- The scope of activity (number of physicians or practices to be established)
- Practice purchase versus equity swap (or other integration strategy)

In addition, working capital for practice operations and physicians' salaries and benefits will be needed.

Capabilities and Resources
If the professional corporation does not have existing practice management resources to draw on, then significant cost is entailed, similar to the start-up of an MSO. This cost may be offset, however, by the practice management capabilities and resources of the acquired practices.

Scope of Activity
The scope of the activity will greatly affect the resources required. Acquiring and managing five or six primary care practices may require $1 million, while 50 practices may require seven to ten times that amount.

Practice Purchase versus Equity Swap

One way to reduce the cost of starting up the trust/professional corporation model is to allow established practitioners to become shareholders in the new corporation, in exchange for tangible and intangible assets of their existing practices (the shared equity model). Although this strategy risks the loss of majority control, it can greatly enhance the chances for long-term success, because the shareholder physicians are more vested in the ultimate success or failure of the practice. Under this approach, a retiring shareholder physician receives an appropriate postretirement payout based on the ownership share of the fair market value of tangible and intangible practice assets. A drawback to shared ownership, however, arises from the requirement that physicians contribute the proportionate share of funding for investment and operating losses.

Other Issues

From a strategic standpoint, the trust/professional corporation model can complement an existing MSO and/or PHO by offering interested physicians the opportunity for full integration through the professional corporation, perhaps while contracting management services through the MSO and/or participating in the PHO. However, over time the trust/professional corporation model can take over those functions.

A separate MSO and/or PHO may make sense for two reasons. First, both can serve a broader and more diverse population of physicians and physician needs. Second, separate funding of a wholly hospital-owned MSO can expand the hospital's control, as well as reduce the issues arising from funding requirements for a trust/professional corporation model that has physician shareholders. A separate MSO will minimize the amount of capital required by the corporation for physician compensation and benefits; the MSO will fund start-up working capital requirements for personnel, supplies, practice site, and equipment purchases.

Because the professional corporation is wholly or partially owned by the hospital, the following conditions must be met. First, practice purchases must be made at fair market value. A full practice appraisal, complying with OIG and IRS guidelines, is required. Similarly, physician compensation must be consistent with industry and market norms. Because of the entity's close relationship to the hospital, it is likely that JCAHO standards and review may apply.

Summary of Trust/Professional Corporation Model

Figure 3-17 summarizes the capabilities and limitations of the trust/professional corporation model. Overall the model appears to be an excellent mechanism for close integration

Figure 3-17. Capabilities and Limitations of the Trust/Professional Corporation Model

Properly executed, the professional corporation:

Does:
- Avoid corporate practice of medicine in some states
- Enable the hospital to purchase practices and employ physicians
- Allow joint physician and indirect hospital ownership of practices
- Have high-cost implications, especially if purchasing practices
- Allow for hospital management and control

Does Not:
- Eliminate private inurement and some fraud and abuse issues (fair market value considerations remain)
- Avoid corporate practice of medicine in all states

between hospital and physicians. However, its application may be limited based on applicable state law regarding corporate practice of medicine. As with all options, qualified legal counsel and analysis are required.

Direct Physician Employment Model

About half of the states in the U.S. do not enforce corporate practice of medicine laws, and in these states the *direct physician employment model* is an attractive option. In areas with high managed care penetration, capitation, and provider integration, physician employment may be an attractive near-term option. In areas in which managed care and hospital–physician integration are not as well developed, physician employment may be a longer-range goal.

Figure 3-18 describes the direct employment model under which physicians become direct employees of the hospital. The hospital bills for all services, manages practice expenses, and controls compensation. Overall, the appeal to the hospital is centralized control over the entire continuum of health care delivery, reduced legal issues related to patient referral flow, and direct investment in physician incomes and practice sites.

An option under this model is to employ a significant portion of medical staff. In Mason City, Iowa, for example, almost all primary care physicians have become employees of the local hospital over the past 10 years. The hospital owns and operates various primary care medical practices and clinics that are within one hour's travel time of Mason City. Only a handful of the city's primary care physicians remain outside this arrangement. With few exceptions, specialists are not a part of this arrangement.

In general, benefits to a hospital under this model can include the following:

- The threat of mass physician defection is reduced significantly.
- The health system can align and control incentive structure to achieve corporate goals.
- Duplication of services between hospital and physicians can be eliminated.
- Patient referrals may be directed to health system resources legally.

Figure 3-18. Typical Direct Employment Model Structure

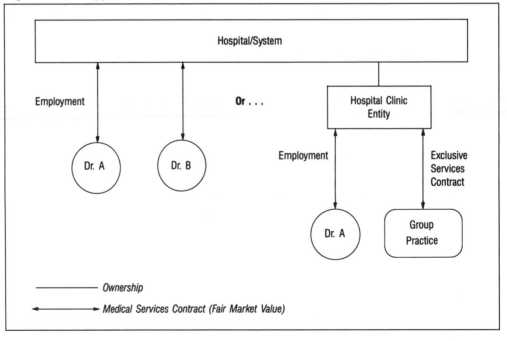

- Health system assets can be allocated toward physician compensation, medical practice facilities, and other needed areas with fewer legal complications.
- The hospital experiences greater protection from fraud and abuse laws.

Physician benefits may include the following:

- Employed physicians may enjoy increased income security and company-paid employee benefits.
- They have many of the advantages of group practice, without needing to invest in facilities and equipment.
- An integrated system allows them increased competitiveness.
- The likelihood of attracting managed care contracts is greater when physicians are employed by the hospital.
- The physicians may gain financially from the sale of their practices (which may or may not include the value of intangible assets).
- They may have access to tax-exempt financing in some health systems.

On the negative side, physicians forgo ownership interests and a certain degree of control and, therefore, entrepreneurial involvement. Once this happens, the potential for business success rests largely with incentive compensation methodologies and the policies and procedures of the health system. Furthermore, in some cases, compensation for intangible assets of an acquired practice may be minimal, and physicians may perceive a loss of retirement funds. Accordingly, structuring benefit and retirement plans for physician employees is critical.

A significant benefit of physician employment arrangements is the attractiveness of this arrangement to managed care payers. Under traditional fee-for-service reimbursement, physicians have been compensated based on production, which has been shown to drive up health care costs. Salaried arrangements, with incentive structures consistent with managed care goals, can be an important marketing advantage for both parties.

Structure and Strategy

The options for direct physician employment can be accomplished in different ways, each with different payment and reimbursement implications. Therefore, careful analysis of reimbursement policies of the major payers is required. From a Medicare standpoint, different cost-based reimbursement is available based on whether services are considered an outpatient division, a clinic, or a faculty practice plan (applicable to teaching hospitals). In addition, there are a variety of special designations that could further enhance or erode compensation. Cost allocation, both for overhead and physician compensation and benefits, can be handled in a variety of ways. Evaluating structural options requires a specific, detailed analysis of reimbursement and cost allocation.

Cost and Capitalization

Research into direct employment arrangements has yielded two observations. One, most institutions feel unable to clearly separate and evaluate the financial performance of clinical physician services from other services. Most often cited are problems with allocating expense, tracking revenue and collections, and evaluating incremental organizational impact from referral business. Second, despite imperfect financial tracking, direct physician employment usually is a "financial loser" until incremental revenue to the hospital and specialists was factored in. The case studies in chapters 9 and 10 illustrate these points well. Additionally, in many cases physician productivity decreases following employment, particularly in salaried relationships, thereby contributing to losses.

The major cost factors depend on the size and number of physicians involved. First, paying physician salaries requires working capital; the health system builds ownership in the accounts receivable asset while paying the physician biweekly for services rendered.

The greater the number of physicians employed, the more working capital is needed for physician compensation and benefits. This is offset by the growth in the accounts receivable asset.

Also, under physician employment by a tax-exempt hospital or entity, the option for equity exchange or sharing in net earnings is not available. Therefore, a policy is needed that addresses whether practices will be purchased. An additional crucial question is whether intangible assets exist and whether they will be purchased. All purchase transactions continue to be guided by the requirement for a fair market valuation, which is due to the fraud and abuse and tax considerations faced by hospitals.

Moreover, the valuation of a practice (based on the IRS's position as of this writing) is directly related to future compensation. It is therefore critical that both compensation and valuation be examined collectively.

Physician Compensation

Physician compensation is typically based on a salary plus bonus. In some areas with minimal managed care penetration, a production-based compensation arrangement is common, or a base salary with the bonus based on overall production.

Physician compensation under managed care is undergoing compression, with the high end and the low end of the physician income range diminishing. This should continue because managed care does not encourage or benefit from the traditional concept of high production (not to be confused with productivity, which is encouraged). Performance is being evaluated based on efficiency measures, patient satisfaction measures, preventive care performance, and overall patient management. All of these incentives have a systemwide impact and align physician rewards with organizational success and managed care goals.

The direct employment model entails a performance review mechanism, including some of the aforementioned measures. This mechanism, in addition to other compensation features, makes this compensation model vastly different from traditional fee-for-service, entrepreneurial practice. Because of this wide cultural and psychological shift, this model is often difficult to implement with established practitioners, particularly with physicians who are not threatened by increasing managed care and capitated reimbursement.

Benefits

Benefits with a tax-exempt organization often provide less opportunity for deferral of income than private practitioners are accustomed to in their practices. Because benefits (especially tax-qualified deferred benefits) effectively provide incentives for lasting employment, employers must develop plans that serve this purpose. At the same time, the employer hospital must view benefits along with other compensation to ensure compliance with tax and other applicable laws. Creating attractive and low-cost plans can serve both parties' goals.

Other Issues

A major political issue often arises in establishing and maintaining positive relationships with nonemployed physicians; for example, as the employment model is introduced, other physicians may feel threatened. Also, the direct employment option requires a great deal of cooperative planning with the medical staff, including identification of environmental threats, organizational vision, and a clear purpose and mandate for the employment arrangement. (See chapter 2 for more on early planning efforts.) Finally, because nonparticipating physicians need reassurance that they are not being left out in the cold, the direct employment option is often accompanied by other services and activities for physicians who desire less-integrated options.

Summary of Direct Physician Employment Model

Figure 3-19 summarizes the direct employment model. This relationship is extremely appealing and well suited to improve performance under managed care. Its biggest

Figure 3-19. Capabilities and Limitations of the Direct Employment Model Structure

Properly executed, direct employment:

Does:

- Maximize hospital control
- Minimize competitive duplication of services
- Enable hospital subsidization of the practice
- Enable referrals to be directed to the employer

Does Not:

- Retain the same entrepreneurial bottom-line incentives for physicians that independent practices offer
- Give physicians any autonomy

challenges lie with the cultural shift required for established physicians and the importance of physician bonus incentive criteria. Despite its drawbacks, this model is very effective in a competitive health care environment and is quickly growing in popularity and physician participation.

Physician Equity Model

The *physician equity model* represents "coming full circle" in the continuum of physician–hospital integration. In essence, physicians are partial or complete owners of a health system entity, fully vested mentally and financially in the practice. Through stock or other equity ownership, physicians share the risk and reward for success in the various entities. As is the case in their private practice, physicians holding equity will be better motivated, more committed, and more closely aligned with organizational goals.

Because of physician ownership, these entities do not qualify for tax-exempt status. Depending on the organizational form selected, the entity itself may be a separate, taxable entity.

This model is represented by organizations such as the Mullikin Medical Group in southern California, whose participants developed a strong, wholly physician-owned integrated health care delivery system. Although a number of long-standing, physician practice–based, fully integrated models exist (such as the Cleveland Clinic, Ochsner Clinic, and Mayo Clinic), these organizations are less-relevant models for emulation because of the long history and highly evolved nature of integrated care delivery associated with these organizations and because their tax-exempt status prevents physician equity ownership. Other variations of the physician equity model exist, such as Pacific Physician Services, a rapidly expanding public company that, through indirect control of an affiliated group practice, employs approximately 200 physicians in the southwestern United States.

A tremendous advantage to wholly physician-owned organizations is that typically they can buy and integrate other medical practices with fewer legal obstacles. As a result, transactions are consummated in two to four months and with minimum legal effort and organizational restructuring.

The biggest problem with the equity model is the capital requirement. As in any group practice, initial investment, growth, and efficiency require capital, which may affect shareholder earnings or dilute an investor's interest. Moreover, an equity model requires physicians to contribute to capital, rather than selling their capital stake as in other models. Thus, other models may provide the potential for a larger up-front buyout of a physician's practice.

57

However, capital for expansion may be available from other sources. For example, to raise needed capital, Mullikin sold 15 percent of Mullikin Management to The Daughters of Charity in St. Louis, which committed to a $50 million investment. As part of the deal, Mullikin will manage several Daughters of Charity IPAs.

Structure

The legal issues and structure of the physician equity model (whose essential elements are depicted in figure 3-20) are much simpler concerns than is the case with other integration models. Organizational relationships are driven largely by business issues. In the case of the Mullikin group, for example, physicians own a share in some or all of its entities.

The parent is the majority owner of both the hospital and the management company. The professional corporation and the IPA enter into contracts for medical services with the management company. All revenues and managed care contracts are held by the parent.

A hospital or health system can participate in a physician equity model in three ways. One way is as an equity participant and business partner, potentially contributing financial resources and business expertise. Another is as a contract inpatient facility. The third mode of participation is as the seller of inpatient or other assets to the physician equity entity.

Cost and Capitalization

Significant investment is required to establish efficient practice sites, a systems and communications infrastructure, and integration of the various constituent practices. Compared to previously discussed models, however, physician equity costs are likely to be lower because of the opportunity to swap equity with newly acquired physicians. In exchange for the practice assets, the physician(s) receive stock or ownership in the group practice and share in profits and losses accordingly.

Figure 3-20. Typical Physician Equity Model Structure

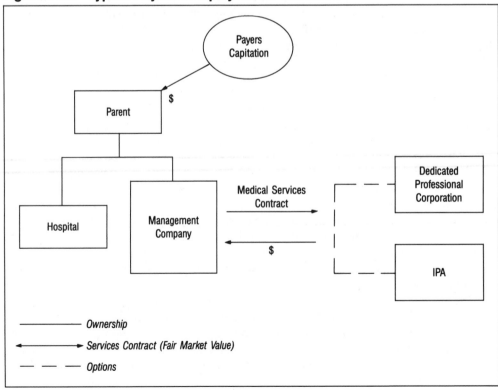

Additional savings are incurred as a result of fewer legal and accounting costs associated with this model. On the negative side, the physician equity model is a taxable entity, and organizational profits are taxed before earnings are allocated to the shareholders.

Typically, there are two funding sources for future growth. One is outside investors—either a large investor such as the Mullikin–Daughters of Charity deal, or the public markets, such as Pacific Physician Services. The second option is retained earnings, which in turn reduces shareholder earnings.

To minimize the draw on precious capital resources, especially important in a rapidly growing system such as Mullikin, physician equity organizations are carefully evaluating their investment options. Often these organizations prefer to contract outside services rather than purchase or develop new services internally.

Operations

A tremendous advantage to the physician equity model is how it lends itself to complete integration of all systems, including development of a single medical record, quality and outcomes tracking across the entire spectrum of care, and ability to understand costs and create profitable package pricing arrangements. This degree of integration is difficult or impossible to achieve in the more fragmented models. Despite the separate organizational entities depicted in figure 3-20, internal divisions are minimized, and the organization functions as a single entity by virtue of common ownership.

To achieve *full* integration, however, the equity model must involve some relationship with an outpatient hospital. If physicians are to acquire a hospital, they must obtain the capital needed to do so. Without this relationship, the equity model has the potential to become nothing more than a large group practice.

Control

In a physician equity model, physicians control the organization. However, a problem often encountered in group practices is instability due to constantly changing (and easily changeable) leadership structure. A key challenge for this arrangement is to create stability for organizational leadership. Strong leadership and consistency of vision is important. In the case of Mullikin, the 12-member board of directors consists of the 6 "founder" directors, who have what amounts to lifetime appointments, and 6 directors elected by the shareholders who serve two-year terms. The selected directors are nominated by the executive committee, which consists of the 6 founder directors.

Compensation

Physician compensation in a physician equity model can come from three sources. First is salary, which is usually based on physician specialty and market factors, with performance criteria for annual increases. At Mullikin, for example, physician salaries are set at the 75th percentile of the Medical Group Management Association's annual compensation survey for a given specialty. In addition, physician employees may receive bonuses based on criteria related to overall organizational goals. Second, income may be derived from shareholder earnings on the appreciation of the equity investment, which are based on overall organizational profit. Finally, physicians may receive payment for management and administrative services. With these payment mechanisms, physicians' direct incentives and performance are easily aligned with the organization's goals.

Other Issues

State insurance requirements regarding capitated risk may dictate that in order to take full risk, including capitation for hospital care, the system may be required to own an inpatient facility. This would enable the organization to subcapitate other hospitals, as well as admit patients to system-owned hospitals. Significant profit can be made through the ability to control and subcapitate hospital care. Doing so, however, also may require that the organization obtain an HMO license and thereby mandate that the organization satisfy applicable capital requirements. This requirement, in turn, increases regulatory costs and the need for additional capital.

Alternatively, if this requirement is not met, the organization would have to contract with hospitals to offer a comprehensive package of services to purchasers. This typically results in the nonintegrated hospital receiving direct capitation from the purchaser, which would reduce profit potential and control of the system. In addition, some states require specific levels of financial reserves on the part of the system in order to take capitated risk.

Summary of Physician Equity Model

The physician equity model can be a superior entity for the cost-efficient and well-organized delivery of comprehensive health care services. Quick movement and integration at relatively lower costs can make it a formidable competitor. Figure 3-21 summarizes key elements.

☐ Business Options

Business options differ from organizational options in that a business option can be applied to most or all of the organizational options identified in the preceding sections. Once the organizational option(s) has been determined, the strategic plan envisioned may help give direction to the business plan related to the following three issues: primary care versus multispecialty group, specialty networks, and group practice without walls.

Primary Care versus Multispecialty Group

The health system can pursue the strategy of primary care–hospital integration or multispecialty–hospital integration. Investment in primary care is common as organizations recognize primary care physicians as an undersupplied commodity in a managed care system. Primary care physicians are the gatekeepers and therefore the controllers of utilization. Because they can make or break the organizations' financial success, they are seen as attractive business partners. Clearly, specialists also need to be involved, whether on a contractual basis or as part of the group, which is the multispecialty strategy option. In most multispecialty organizations, primary care physicians gain by having some expenses offset by the financial contribution of the specialists. Therefore, this arrangement can be attractive to the primary care physicians. In return, the specialists have the security of an internal referral stream.

Figure 3-21. Capabilities and Limitations of the Physician Equity Model Structure

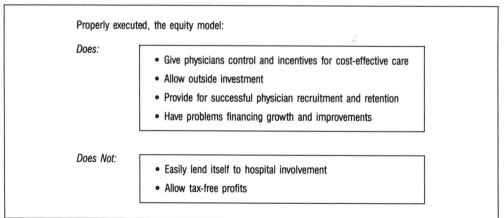

Properly executed, the equity model:

Does:
- Give physicians control and incentives for cost-effective care
- Allow outside investment
- Provide for successful physician recruitment and retention
- Have problems financing growth and improvements

Does Not:
- Easily lend itself to hospital involvement
- Allow tax-free profits

Specialty Networks

Another strategic option pursued by health care organizations is integration of a single specialty group into the organization. This integration is usually driven by one of three situations. Either the locale holds little attraction for specialist recruitment, or the hospital is attempting to establish or bolster a center of excellence, or a single-specialty group forms to bid on sub-capitation arrangements for that specialty. A *center of excellence* is a highly marketed clinical service, such as a cancer center, women's health center, business health clinic, heart institute, sports medicine clinic, or other such specialty niches. In these situations, most of the previously identified organizational models could be used to recruit and retain targeted physicians—with the possible exception of the foundation model and the physician equity model, both of which tend to be larger-scale undertakings.

Group Practice without Walls (GPWW)

A great deal of the controversy over GPWWs is a result of the ambiguity surrounding their definition. The GPWW is not an organizational structure among hospitals and physicians, but rather a business concept applied to a variety of organizational and ownership models.

The GPWW is an arrangement whereby a number of solo physicians or small practices combine their resources into a single professional corporation. Certain operations and functions are centralized, such as billing, managed care contracting, personnel, accounting, and marketing. The physicians continue to operate out of a variety of separate locations, maintaining independent practice sites and allocating site-specific costs to the physician(s) practicing at that site. Participants gain the efficiency and clout of a combined group practice while maintaining autonomy and the financial incentives of their practice production and expenses. Cost of centralized services are shared as mutually agreed.

In the context of hospital–physician integration, the GPWW is implemented under the hospital practice site and assets option, the MSO option, the foundation model, the trust/professional corporation model, and the equity model. The characteristic common to all these relationships is that physicians and their practices are integrated into a single professional corporation which, with varying levels of hospital involvement, attempt to gain economies of scale and improved volume and revenue performance through combined negotiation.

Occasionally a GPWW relationship suffers from unrealistic expectations. Because most group practices are managed as a going concern, continued investment in efficiency and growth requires retention of earnings. In today's health care market, management requirements are also increasing. As a result of these two factors, group practice overhead may not be reduced and in fact may increase. If the future financial needs of the group are not understood up front and expectations set accordingly, the group can suffer serious near-term setbacks.

Overall, the GPWW concept is an attractive and viable arrangement for physicians motivated by continued autonomy but requiring certain benefits of group practice. The usefulness of this vehicle, however, wanes with significant increase in capitated business and the reduction of production-oriented incentives. Enhanced financial performance can be achieved by consolidation of practice sites and operations. Implementation of a GPWW is often an incremental step toward greater and more economical integration.

☐ Conclusion

As demonstrated throughout this chapter, the choice or organizational structure is driven by a variety of factors. Increasingly, however, hospital administrators are promoting a multitiered strategy that involves the concurrent implementation of multiple organizational structures to achieve integration.

To maximize the pace toward integration—as well as hedge administrative bets—administrators can embrace a multi-integration strategy as a logical and practical approach. This strategy allows physicians to be involved with the hospital in a number of ways and, as trust and management capabilities develop, steps up movement toward greater integration.

Chapter 4
Key Business Issues

The process of structuring a hospital–physician integration can be an extremely complicated undertaking. Aside from routine business issues (such as cost-efficiency, delivery of a marketable product or service, meeting consumer demand, and the like), a variety of legal, tax, and political implications must be factored into affiliation negotiations. The outcome is more than a business deal; it is a long-term relationship that must grow, evolve, and accommodate diverse needs in a sometimes adversarial environment. When conflict and discord surface, the business relationship must be capable of withstanding the stress.

Chapter 3 identified the variety of integration models available and, to some extent, the accompanying business considerations unique to each model. This chapter will further detail key business issues that are common to most hospital–physician affiliations and applicable to the range of organizational models described in chapter 3.

Four broad categories of business elements will be covered: financial terms between parties, other major cost factors, political issues, and management and operational considerations. Financial terms between parties center primarily on practice value and purchase, physician compensation, and ancillary services. Other cost factors relate to the manner in which practice equity is attained, the cost of operations, and the growth factor. Political issues include external changes in health care financing (fee for service, capitated payment, managed care) and prioritization of primary care and specialized care. Finally, management and operational questions link the effect of integration on physician autonomy, control, and decision making.

☐ Financial Terms between Parties

The following sections outline common methodologies and rationales for arriving at practice value and physician compensation. Negotiation of ancillary services is discussed separately, although it can affect both the appraisal of practice value and the terms of physician compensation.

Practice Value and Purchase

Integration between hospital and physician involves practice valuation and purchase, in whole or part, in organizational models such as MSOs, foundations, trusts, professional corporations, direct employment, and equity models. Valuation can relate to some or all practice assets. Sometimes assets are valued and purchased up front; if value is not assigned immediately, the parties at least agree to a valuation methodology to be applied at a later specified time. In certain cases, the collaborative entity exchanges stock for the value of the practice. In all cases, however, valuation methods and rationale become key components of the analysis.

As hospitals and group practices design their networks and move forward with integration efforts, appraisal accuracy becomes crucial. The valuation process is triggered by different circumstances, including the following:

- Mergers or acquisitions
- Buy or sell agreements
- New associate employment contracts
- Physician's departure or retirement payout
- Physician's divorce or death
- Hospital-sponsored group practice development

Regardless of the motives involved, a good valuation process keeps three objectives in focus: (1) relations between the integrative parties should be enhanced, (2) legal ramifications should be minimized, and (3) the transaction should be positioned for tax advantages. In assigning a practice value, both the physician's perspective and the hospital's perspective should be kept in mind.

Physician Perspective

The new physician's perception of practice value has expanded over the past decade or so. Physicians already in practice are seeing more patients in an effort to offset reimbursement declines, thus reducing available patient volume for new practitioners. Also, enormous start-up costs and administrative requirements make starting a solo practice impractical for new physicians. The option to buy an existing practice from a retiring physician, in a desirable location with an established patient base, is attractive from the viewpoint of avoiding the high costs and risks associated with new practice start-up. A second option is for the physician to become an employee of a group practice, HMO, or similar entity, which provides stability, guaranteed income, regular hours, and increased flexibility. Whether the physician decides to purchase a practice or buy into an established one, practice valuation is usually a part of the process.

Hospital Perspective

Increased government involvement and scrutiny of hospital–physician transactions have pressed hospitals to substantiate assistance to physicians. Physician bidding wars have been replaced with careful analysis of physician practices due to uncertainty in the industry regarding the value of intangibles. As emphasized in chapter 3, documentation of fair market value transactions is essential.

Although many methods exist for obtaining a range of value (as discussed in the following subsections), some can be justified more readily than others. Whichever methods are used ultimately, it is important to focus on examining the fair market value of the practice and maintaining an arm's-length transaction. Toward this end, many hospitals and medical groups seek experienced outside advisers in their appraisal efforts.

Methods of Practice Valuation

Because each appraisal method examines different aspects of a practice, no two methods will yield identical results. Therefore, several techniques must be used to arrive at a reasonable *range of value*. In fact, the 1994 IRS Continuing Professional Education Technical Instruction Program suggests that the use of "all recognized approaches for estimating the value of a going concern" is desirable.[1] However, it is important to note that common methods used to appraise other businesses may be unsuitable for valuing a medical practice.

Practice valuations can be applied to specific practice assets—including hard assets, accounts receivable, and intangibles—or to the practice as a whole. In the latter case, valuation is often referred to as *business enterprise value* (discussed later in the chapter) and includes stock valuations.

Hard Assets

The value assigned to hard assets is based on one of four methods: book value, modified book value, replacement value, and fair market value. *Book value* reflects the value of an asset as it appears on the practice balance sheet. In other words, the book value is the original purchase price less accumulated depreciation.

Modified book value, a more popular variation of the book value method, considers the original purchase price of the assets and then applies straight-line depreciation based on the average useful life of each item. For instance, assume that a piece of equipment purchased three years ago for $1,000 has an estimated useful life of five years. Under the modified book value method, the item has a current value of $400 as calculated in the following equation:

$$\$1,000 - (\$1,000 \times \tfrac{3}{5}) = \$400$$

A valuable resource for determining estimated useful life is the book *Estimated Useful Lives of Depreciable Hospital Assets*, 1993 edition, published by American Hospital Publishing, Inc. Estimated useful lives range from 3 to 15 years. One drawback to this method is that estimated life may be underestimated (too short), and assets may have a residual value after the term of the estimated life.

The last two valuation methods require the determination of current market values. *Replacement value* reflects the amount required to replace each asset at current prices. *Fair market value* usually incorporates estimates from experienced appraisers, salespeople, and equipment dealers to determine a price the used practice assets would command on the open market. The fair market value approach may incorporate a combination of well-reasoned methods.

Certain items—artwork, for example—should be excluded from valuation. This is because, although they may have minimal monetary value to an appraiser, they may be priceless to the physician who owns them. Typically, such assets have highly variable and speculative values.

Accounts Receivable

The status of accounts receivable may reflect the level of efficiency in business operations. Valuation, then, should be based on the best possible estimate of collectibility. These accounts also can be evaluated based on the practice specialty, age, and payer mix. Because of variability in collection performance, it may be easier to allow the seller to collect the revenue stream from pretransaction accounts receivable rather than attempt to assign a value. This approach can avoid the cost involved with developing an accurate estimate of value and/or the discord that can arise when negotiating a purchase price.

Intangibles

Although intangibles is usually the largest and most important component of valuation, it is also the most subjective and variable. Intangibles include location, size of patient base, practice reputation, established contracts, assembled workforce, and so forth. Practices capable of transferring intangibles to a successor (primary care, for example) will yield higher values. A variety of tax and legal issues arise when considering intangibles and whether they can be purchased, and these issues are addressed in chapter 5.

The value of a going concern (going-concern value) can be estimated using income approaches, market approaches, and cost approaches. The IRS has indicated that the income approaches appear to be most relevant because they incorporate the capitalization of excess earnings method and the discounted future cash flow method.[2] Market approaches such as the comparable sale method, the subjective composite rating approach, and the blended industry "rule of thumb" are also popular. The "rule-of-thumb" methods, although widely reported, are generally not reliable indicators, particularly on a stand-alone basis, and are therefore not recommended.

In the *capitalization of excess earnings approach,* a weighted average of the physician's net income for a minimum of three years is calculated. This average is then compared to a weighted average compensation figure for a physician employed in the same specialty in that geographic area. The difference between the two is the excess earnings of the practice. Applying a capitalization rate based on risk and other factors yields the value of the practice intangibles. Adding the fair market value for practice hard assets produces the practice valuation.[3]

This excess earnings method is used throughout the industry and is identified by the IRS as an applicable method of valuing practice intangibles.[4,5] However, the approach can understate or overstate the value of intangibles because it does not factor in the marketability of practice assets. In addition, there is subjectivity involved in determining a capitalization rate, and this can yield a skewed value.

The method used most often to identify the full business enterprise value of a practice is the *discounted cash flow approach,* which contemplates the complete value of the practice including practice assets, hard assets, accounts receivable, and intangibles. Typically it does not take into account cash, checking account balances, and certain practice liabilities. Liabilities can be considered in those situations where acquisition or transfer of practice stock is involved.

This methodology is based on the principle of anticipation, that is, what a buyer can expect in terms of future benefit. It reflects those forces likely to affect future revenues, expenses, and earnings of a practice. Future practice revenues are estimated based on anticipated volume and reimbursement changes. From these numbers, estimated expenses are deducted. Expenses should include a reasonable level of compensation for an employed physician (or physician group) based on averages for comparable physicians in that geographic area and on practice workload. The result is the net income to be discounted back to present-day value by applying an appropriate discount rate that factors in the risk associated with projections and practice performance. The net result of this calculation is the total present value of the practice.

The discounted cash flow approach is useful in determining a range of value. However, because the focus is on profits and cash flow, and not on specific assets, and because it relies on analysis of uncertain future events, this approach is speculative. Therefore, it should be used in combination with other valuation methodologies.

The excess earnings approach and the discounted cash flow both are emphasized by the IRS. In fact, Revenue Ruling 76-91 mandates use of the excess earnings approach despite the IRS's pronouncement that it is "inadequate" (Revenue Ruling 68-609).[6] Revenue Ruling 59-60 is regarded as the standard framework within which a valuation is performed.[7] Figure 4-1 lists highlights of this ruling and the considerations a valuation must address.

The *comparable sale method* arrives at practice worth by comparing an estimate to the average purchase price of other practice intangible assets of the same specialty. Net revenues are multiplied by the average "goodwill" percentage (historical sale prices for intangibles in that specialty divided by practice annual collections) to obtain a value for the practice intangibles. Hard assets and accounts receivable are later added to identify total practice value.

The benefit of this method is that it applies the financial performance of the subject practice to an actual market pricing for intangibles. It is important, however, to analyze

Figure 4-1. Revenue Ruling 59-60: Framework for Practice Valuation

Over the past 30 years, the IRS has issued several revenue rulings relating to business valuation. Although these rulings themselves are not law, they do present the IRS's position on tax matters related to the valuation of business and business interests. The IRS has recently scrutinized fraud and abuse activity with respect to medical practice purchase. This has focused appraisers' attention to these rulings as *the* framework upon which to build a credible valuation.

The following outlines some of the key components of Revenue Ruling 59-60. Released in 1959 and updated in 1968 by Revenue Ruling 68-609, it is the standard by which valuations of closely held businesses are performed.

Closely held businesses are corporations whose shares are owned by a limited number of stockholders or, in many cases, one individual. Because buying and selling of these businesses takes place infrequently, there is no established market. As a result, these sales seldom reflect all of the elements of a "fair market value" transaction. The determination of fair market value will therefore depend upon the circumstances in each case.

A sound valuation will be based upon all the relevant facts, but the elements of common sense, informed judgement, and reasonableness must enter into the process of weighing those facts and determining their aggregate significance.

In determining fair market value of medical practices, the following items must be considered:

- Going concern status of the practice
- Nature of the practice and the history of the enterprise from its inception
- Current and historical financial condition of the practice, analysis of operating ratios, and trends of financial results
- Earnings capacity of the practice
- Historical earnings and factors that affect earnings, such as competitive position, markets, and market penetration
- Successor management of the practice
- General economic outlook and the conditions and outlook of the health care industry
- Similar sales of medical practices in same or similar specialty and geographic area

The valuation of closely held businesses, like medical practices, entails the consideration of all the relevant factors mentioned above. Depending upon the circumstances in each case, certain factors may carry more weight than others because of the nature of the particular medical practice.

Source: Revenue Ruling 59-60, 1959-1, C.B. 237.

the largest possible number of comparable market transactions in order to use this method. Comparable sale pricing based on one to three comparables can yield an inappropriate result. The principal shortcoming of the comparable sale method is that good comparative sales data can be difficult to obtain. Generally speaking, solid information is available to support the valuation of primary care practices but is more limited for specialty practices.

The *subjective composite rating approach* compares the intangible characteristics of a medical practice to those of an average practice within that specialty, using comparative statistics from multiple sources, such as the AMA and the MGMA (Medical Group Management Association), as well as direct experience with other similar practices. Gross receipts, profitability, location, staffing, competition, payer mix, and transferability, among other factors, are examined. The result is a multiplier that is applied to the comparable sale value for intangibles, thus increasing or decreasing the value yielded by the comparable sale valuation. Hard assets and accounts receivable are then added in, resulting in the total practice value.

This method takes into account practice characteristics not normally considered in other methodologies and rates the practice relative to an average performance for that specialty according to the practice's efficiency, attractiveness, transferability, reputation, and demographics. A shortcoming is the subjective nature of the approach—some ratings represent nothing more than the appraiser's opinion based on personal experience with other practices and knowledge of the market.

The *blended industry rule-of-thumb method* considers several individual formulas that, with minor variation, value the hard assets, accounts receivable, and clinical aspects of the practice or its intangibles. Formulas typically used have appeared in industry journals such as *Medical Economics, Physician's Management,* and *Money Management.* The results of these formulas can be averaged, excluding outliers, to obtain an estimate of value based on published, albeit unsophisticated and unsubstantiated, approaches. Although inadequate as a stand-alone method, the blended industry approach ties in a variety of information sources that may be familiar to the buying and/or selling physician. Given the circulation of the preceding publications, many transactions have been influenced by these published methodologies and therefore can be included in market approaches.

Other Considerations

The process of valuation is lengthy and subject to inaccuracy without close attention to detail. When comparing a subject practice's elements to national and regional averages, valuation analysts must match "apples to apples." Also, because practice transition is a critical period, the length of time the selling physician is expected to remain on board to facilitate transition is another key consideration. Increased physician cooperation may mean increased value, because more patients are likely to remain with the practice, but paying two physician salaries may decrease "excess earnings," thereby reducing the value. Other issues include transferability of software, quality of practice staff, revenue sources, managed care contracts, and coding.

Finally, after several valuation approaches have been applied and evaluated and a range of value determined, the question will remain: At what price will the seller sell and at what price will the buyer buy? Only a good sense of the market and knowledge of both buyer and seller will help determine a range of value that will satisfy both parties.

Allocation of Value

Upon determination of practice value, the next issue is how it will be allocated among assets. From both the buyer's and seller's perspective, it is desirable to maximize the after-tax impact of the transaction. The purchaser is interested in purchasing depreciable assets so as to maximize the allocation to hard assets, patient records, and payment for a noncompete covenant. Over the past six years, the selling physician was generally indifferent as to how the purchase price was allocated because tax treatment remained consistent between ordinary income and capital gains. However, with the 1993 change in tax law, capital gains will be taxed at a lower rate, generally prompting the seller to maximize the value attributed to practice intangibles (goodwill, assembled workforce, payer contracts, location, and so forth), which are taxable at the lower capital gains rate. The ideal value allocation of the buyer, from a tax standpoint, is therefore at odds with the ideal allocation for the seller. A retiring physician may wish to receive payment after retirement, over time, plus interest, to take advantage of a lower tax rate. Because the economics of transactions depend on individual circumstances, it is strongly recommended that both parties seek expert legal and tax advice to maximize economic advantages of the deal.

Physician Compensation

Physician compensation, along with practice valuation and control, is a key element in the hospital–physician integration process. Traditionally, physicians have had a direct link between services performed and financial remuneration, consistent with the culture of independent practice and entrepreneurship. With the advent of capitation and managed care, the definition of *services performed* has been expanded to include the responsible management of fixed resources. *Fixed resources* refers to prepaid revenues for patient care (capitation) and maximization of existing medical, technological, and clerical resources. Identifying organizational goals and creating compensation incentives that are consistent with those goals are critical to future success.

Physicians can receive compensation for medical services, administrative services, or shareholder return on investment. Some integrated entities allow for physicians to receive a combination of the three. From a business standpoint, compensation becomes the single most powerful tool to achieve organizational goals and success. However, Medicare fraud and abuse and private inurement restrictions weigh heavily on the determination of compensation methodologies and amounts.

Compensation methods are affected by the status of the physician in the integrated relationship. Figure 4-2 identifies the relationship options that reflect an increasing level of integration, from contractor to shareholder status. These categories are not mutually exclusive; that is, a physician can be both an employee and a shareholder, although shareholder status reflects a more integrated relationship than nonshareholder status. The physician's integration status strongly affects compensation mechanisms and their relative risk, as shown in figure 4-3. Higher levels of integration often exhibit more shared risk–reward compensation mechanisms. The mechanisms identified in figure 4-3 are summarized briefly in the following sections.

Figure 4-2. Levels of Physician Integration

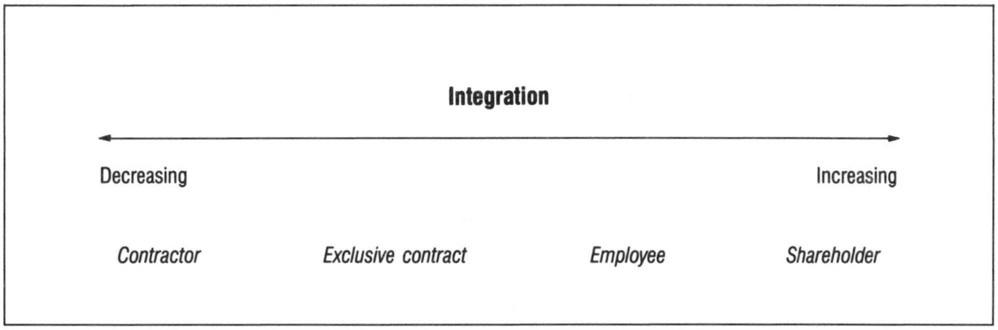

Integration

Decreasing ←――――――――――――――――――――――→ Increasing

Contractor   Exclusive contract   Employee   Shareholder

Figure 4-3. Common Individual Physician Compensation Mechanisms

Least Risk–Reward Influence

Salary

Salary plus bonus

Production — percent of revenue (capitation, production, or both)

Managed care pools/withholds

Bottom line
- Revenue and expense allocation
- True bottom line

Full capitation

Most Risk–Reward

Other Criteria/Factors
- Seniority
- Buy-in/payout adjustments
- Cash versus accrual (asset ownership implications)
- Administrative compensation

Salary

A straight salary appeals to some physicians, particularly younger physicians who may be unable or unwilling to take on significant financial risk (perhaps because of outstanding educational loans or heavy family commitments). However, straight salary, although it carries less risk, runs counter to the entrepreneurial spirit that is a tradition in medical practice; this relationship also restricts physician autonomy. Salaried physicians typically make no investment in the professional corporation. In fact, the corporation invests working capital by funding the lag between actual collections generated by the physician and the timing of the physician's initial paychecks. In this way, the business risk is borne entirely by the organization. As a result, the physician has no claim to individual accounts receivable.

Salary Plus Bonus

Traditional fee-for-service medical practices allocated bonuses based on physician production (volume and/or collections). Under managed care, however, this has changed. Figure 4-4 identifies a number of common bonus criteria under traditional fee for service and managed care. Many large managed care organizations, such as Kaiser and U.S. Healthcare, are still experimenting with different bonus criteria and their relative effectiveness in helping an organization achieve its goals. (See figure 4-5.)

Figure 4-4. Common Bonus Criteria

Traditional Fee for Service
- Revenue production
- Patient volume
- Profit sharing

Managed Care/Capitation
- Withhold pools/profit sharing
  —Specialist utilization
  —Inpatient utilization
  —ER utilization
- Efficiency
- Adherence to protocols
- Patient satisfaction, wait time
- Preventive measures (for example, immunizations)
- Peer review
- Profit sharing

Figure 4-5. Sample Quality-Based Incentives

What It Takes to Be Rated a Good Doctor

Here are some of the more than 20 quality standards used by U.S. Healthcare Inc. to determine what level of incentive payments family practitioners, pediatricians, and internists will receive on delivering high-quality medical care.

- How easy is it to make appointments for checkups?
- How long is the waiting time in a doctor's office?
- How much personal concern does a doctor show for patients?
- How readily can patients obtain follow-up test results?
- Would patients recommend their doctor to others?
- Do doctors provide regular immunizations for children? Breast cancer checks for women? Colon cancer checks for men?
- What percentage of a doctor's patients transfer to another physician's care each year?

Note: Answers to the first five questions are based on patient responses to questionnaires. Answers to the last two questions are based on examination of doctors' medical records and U.S. Healthcare's internal data.

Source: Wall Street Journal, Jan. 25, 1993, p. B1.

Production

Production-based compensation represents a higher risk–reward level. Often represented as a percentage of revenue, traditionally this percentage of production (collections) was attributed to the individual physician. An important caveat here is that, under cash basis accounting, the "percent of revenue" production arrangements will yield extremely low compensation at the outset (in noncapitated settings). This is because of the accounts receivable lag, that is, the time lapse between performance of service and collection of revenue. If physicians are paid based on a percentage of cash collections, it follows that they would have a claim on a portion of the outstanding accounts receivable relative to their individual production, calculated by applying the percentage of cash collections received as compensation to the collectible value of the outstanding accounts receivable upon departure. Even a nonshareholder physician logically would be entitled to this compensation upon departure from the practice.

Under capitation, production may be interpreted as the payment per member per month (PMPM) times the number of covered lives. Revenue, however, is determined contractually, and "production" is determined by the number of members assigned to the physician.

Managed Care Pools/Withholds

By participating in managed care withholds, physicians increase their level of risk and potential return. Typically, referring physicians benefit from withhold pools if they can minimize the cost and expenditure associated with referrals outside the entity. These mechanisms carry risk for the physicians because a portion of their normal compensation is "withheld" as a contingency fund should the allocated funds for specialists or hospitalization services be exceeded. The "reward" is triggered if the referring physician's collective cost of outside referrals to specialists and hospitals is less than the funds allocated, resulting in the excess funds being shared back to that physician. In this fashion, referring physicians are influenced by financial incentive to promote cost-effective care of the patient population.

The maximum physician benefit is derived from a healthy population, which results in minimal need for medical resources of any type. Because prepaid services yield significant benefit to the physician group taking the capitation, the logical extension of capitated care is to maximize preventive services and maintain optimal health among the population.

Bottom Line

Bottom-line compensation can apply to a physician having employee, contractor, or shareholder status. Various calculations may create revenue and expense allocations such that ultimate compensation is the difference between allocated revenues and expenses. The key here becomes allocation of expenses. Capital expenses, as well as operating expenses, may be identified as an overhead expense as well as compensation for certain physicians' administrative services. In addition, outside management companies, and perhaps certain shareholders, may receive compensation through an expense allocation. Ultimately, the shareholder bears the impact of the final bottom line—after various physician compensation calculations—whether it is a gain or a loss.

A key issue in bottom-line compensation, particularly if the physician is not a shareholder, is the allocation of capital investment. In practices that use cash basis accounting, if a major capital expenditure is made, the bottom line is negative. Nonshareholder physicians compensated based on the bottom line would be negatively affected by a capital expense allocation, but they would have no increased equity to offset the reduction in compensation. This issue must be taken into account; otherwise, over time, nonshareholder physicians will become dissatisfied with the practice arrangement.

Full Capitation

Full capitation involves maximum risk, not just for practice performance but for the entire spectrum of health care costs associated with the assigned population. Under full capitation, the physician bears the risk (and cost) for all needed health care services, including specialist care and sometimes inpatient services. The physician would still bear the risks associated with previously discussed compensation methodologies. Because of the high level of risk involved, full capitation is rarely used for individual physician compensation. Rather, it is typically a payment mechanism for a provider group (where risk is shared by the entire group), within which the aforementioned individual compensation methods are applied.

Other Compensation Factors

A number of other components and issues may be factored into physician compensation. For example, a new recruit may be employed on a production or bottom-line compensation basis but initially is guaranteed a base salary, perhaps with a bonus. This may be necessary due to competition for new recruits in certain specialties; this strategy would enable the employer to extend an attractive, low-risk offer.

An adjustment to compensation may be made for practice "buy-in" or "payout." In this scenario, compensation may be calculated by uniform methods but reduced to enable physicians to become equity participants, or shareholders, in the practice. The amount of buy-in required usually is established by a practice valuation and is contributed to the group as a reduction in compensation over several years. Conversely, upon retirement physicians may receive a payout, or deferred compensation, according to the same practice valuation methodology. It is not uncommon, however, for practices to overlook this rationale for buy-ins and payouts.

Additional compensation may be factored in for seniority or administrative services. This is usually driven by the organization's bylaws and is subject to change by shareholder vote.

A variety of issues are connected to the method of accounting. *Cash accounting,* typical in many practices, particularly smaller groups, can greatly affect compensation during years of significant investment. *Accrual accounting* has the effect of distributing these investments over time. Care must be taken to avoid inappropriate and inadvertent accounting impact on the welfare of physician employees and shareholders.

Employee Benefit Plans

The employee benefit issue is a complex and potentially costly aspect of the integration process. Recruitment and retention of key doctors will force health care systems to become more creative in their benefit offerings. The design of the plans will likely be compared to competitive alternatives from hospitals, HMOs, and private practices, among others. Hospital benefit plans often fall short of physician expectations. For this reason, the employee benefits policy should be addressed thoroughly and early in the process.

Benefit plans include, but are not imited to, the following offerings:

- Qualified retirement plans, such as pension plans, profit-sharing plans, and 401(K) plans
- Welfare plans, such as medical and life insurance plans
- Nonqualified retirement plans, such as excess benefit and deferred compensation or deferred bonus plans
- Severance and fringe benefit plans

Benefit issues affect the health system's ability to offer competitive recruiting packages to highly sought-after primary care physicians and provide existing key practitioners with benefits comparable to those found in private practices. Benefit plans will be a great concern for successful practicing physicians. The impact of benefit changes on practicing physicians should be identified in detail early in the recruitment process and be factored into financial discussions.

In recent years many physicians have abandoned regular pension plans, generally the best tax-deferral plans for mature physicians, because of new contribution limits. The

1993 tax law imposed substantial limits on high-income individuals by reducing the qualified deferral capability from $235,840 in 1993 to $150,000 in 1994. This 35 percent reduction in future benefits, along with higher marginal tax rates, exemption phaseouts, and other new tax rules, effectively increased taxes to physicians.

If benefits are constrained by the hospital organization, the physicians' contributions cannot exceed the discrimination boundaries of the hospital employees. For example, a tax-deferred annuity (TDA) plan allows a $9,500 maximum contribution under a not-for-profit hospital plan. This maximum would be unappealing to a physician who annually invests $30,000 in a money purchase and profit-sharing plan.

The vehicles of the policies should also be examined. For example, are the investments in the various TDA offerings competitive? Does the disability company have a high denial rate, and is it financially viable? These questions may be asked by physicians and their representatives and therefore ought to be considered in advance.

If the physicians affiliate under a not-for-profit organizational structure, it severely limits the ability to offer nonqualified deferred-compensation arrangements. Qualified and nondeferred plans are usually grouped together. Under competitive conditions the not-for-profit physician organizations are at a disadvantage for recruitment in comparison to for-profit entities.

The controlled group, affiliated service group, and leased employee rules also raise concerns for physicians and hospitals anticipating a hospital affiliation or similar affiliation. If a medical group has an affiliation with a hospital or other entity, the hospital and medical group may be treated as a single employer for purposes of meeting the nondiscrimination tests for retirement plans. The single-employer determination will occur if the medical group and the hospital are members of the same "controlled group" or "affiliated service group." Other regulations regarding "leased employees" may require that employees of the hospital or other entity who perform services for the medical group be treated as employees of the medical group for purposes of determining whether the benefit plans of the medical group are eligible for favorable tax treatment.

Another common benefits issue is disability insurance. If the physician is to be included under the hospital's benefits, it must be recognized that many group hospital plans have insufficient disability coverage. Physician employees will be partially uncovered.

There are both legal and business issues to consider when deciding whether to merge or terminate retirement plans among groups. If a plan is terminated, for example, all the benefits accrued as of the final date must be made 100 percent vested. This means the physician would need to have the necessary cash available. For these reasons and others, it is important to retain a knowledgeable benefits expert and an attorney who specializes in benefits.

Control of Compensation

An increasingly popular business arrangement is to structure the physician–hospital integration in such a way as to establish a payment mechanism for the physicians as a group. In turn the group determines compensation among individual physicians. In larger groups, compensation may be subdivided into payment mechanisms for individual departments, whose department leaders in turn set up individual physician compensation arrangements. An advantage is that the hospital, health system, and other lay entities are removed from the physician compensation issue, which is a hotbed of controversy in any group practice. Two significant disadvantages are that the organization loses control of individual incentives and that organizational goals may not be reflected in individual physicians' compensation arrangements. Both problems ultimately could be to the detriment of the entire organization and result in reduced cost-effectiveness and loss of market competitiveness.

A common problem in group practices and in teaching/faculty practice plan settings is dissention among departmental "fiefdoms," which typically are dominated by specialists. The trend toward primary care practices under managed care and health care reform is reversing this situation.

Ancillary Services

The profit from ancillary services is usually a substantial benefit to larger group practices. Therefore, how service benefits are allocated within an integrated relationship can be a major negotiation point.

Allocation of ancillary service revenue also has legal ramifications. Care must be taken, for example, to avoid "payment for patient referral," where physicians receive direct payment for referrals made to ancillary services. However, this practice may be less problematic for a large group practice.

Group Practice Options

Physicians wrestle with the issue of allocating ancillary revenues within the group. Generally three options are available. Assume, for example, that a 15-member multispecialty practice has an EKG unit, echocardiogram and treadmill, and a single cardiologist who performs all related services. An option in this scenario is for the cardiologist to derive full benefit from the volume of associated ancillary services and tests performed by him or her.

A second option allocates revenues to a specific site, or a subset of physicians in the larger group. In this case the parent practice may be made up of multiple sites, each with its own X-ray facility, laboratory, and EKG unit. The financial benefits, or profit from services, are allocated only to the bottom line of physicians at the one practice site. An additional determination needs to be made as to whether physicians split the benefit evenly, in proportion to volume or revenue, or apply it as a reduction to overhead expense.

The third option is to allocate the benefit of ancillary services broadly across all physicians in a group practice. This is accomplished as a reduction, or an offset to group overhead expenses. In larger and more complicated group settings a combination of these three options may be used.

Integrated Relationship Options

How the hospital is involved in the affiliation adds another layer of options. One is to match the benefit derived from ancillary services to investment in the service. Another is to structure formalized hospital–physician joint ventures, relationships that are regulated heavily by the Stark Bill (discussed in chapter 5). Other options include the following:

- The hospital receives the full financial benefit.
- The physicians receive the full financial benefit.
- The parties benefit jointly from these services.

A key business (and legal) principle is that the benefit derived should be proportionate to the level of investment (risk) in the business. This investment can be in the form of funding capital costs for the equipment, past marketing and development efforts, and working capital investment over time. For existing services, it is easiest to keep the financial benefit with the entity that made the initial investment.

The business plan, however, may call for a change in investment and performance of these services. For example:

- Consolidation of ancillary services exclusively at the hospital
- Enhancement or development of new ancillary services at the practice site(s) in accordance with community needs
- Hospital purchase of practice ancillary services and continued practice site operation as an extension of hospital outpatient services

A change in ownership would require valuation and purchase of all or a portion of the value of the ancillary service business(es).

In less integrated relationships, such as an MSO, physicians may give up or sell specific hard assets and ancillary service business to the hospital MSO. In this case, there would be valuation and purchase of some or all aspects of the ancillary business, or opportunity for the physicians to continue to derive financial benefit from the business. Sometimes this arrangement is structured as a *revenue guarantee,* that is, a guaranteed minimum percentage of collections paid the physicians as compensation, based on their prior overhead and take-home compensation percentage, with ancillary services included.

In addition to financial issues between the negotiating parties, there are reimbursement issues associated with these options. Operating the services as a hospital extension can enhance or reduce reimbursement. In a capitated setting, however, ancillary services become cost centers and must be evaluated based on their contribution to efficiency and patient convenience as well as the needs of the overall provider network.

The deal between hospital and physicians may not be dictated primarily by business issues. Often physicians may maintain ancillary services, including associated revenues, even though these services could be delivered efficiently and cost-effectively in the hospital's centralized site. These trade-offs may be addressed over time, as capitation increases and the magnitude of incremental revenue diminishes.

A related issue is treatment of revenues from the billing of allied professionals such as nurses, physical therapists, midwives, and various physician extenders. These revenues may be allocated to each allied professional as part of the compensation package or to specific departments. Another option is for the revenues to be reflected as a reduction in overhead, either for a specific site or for the overall organization.

The issue of ancillary services and allied professionals is simplified in a capitated setting. Under capitation, separate revenue and billing for services are largely eliminated; the organizational goal is to provide ancillary services as efficiently and cost-effectively as possible while maximizing the population's health status. For this reason, it is not uncommon to see an increase in preventive screening and associated ancillary services (such as mammography and certain laboratory tests) under capitation.

Treatment of revenues from ancillary services, then, can be a major negotiation point in areas that remain largely fee for service, and, because of the options and subjectivity in dealing with this issue, allocation is a key business element in tailoring an overall financial impact of the affiliation in a way that will meet the needs of the various parties. Ancillary services can be moved from one site or entity to another, or various investment options can be considered so as to achieve the desired financial outcome.

☐ Other Critical Cost Factors

A key cost factor depends on whether a collaborative entity will "make," "buy," or "swap" equity for medical practices. One alternative to the high cost of purchasing practices and starting new ones is shared equity, through which physicians exchange specified assets for ownership in the new entity.

Another issue is cost of operations and infrastructure. Cost of operations may not be limited to ordinary practice operating expenses. If a large-scale enterprise is being established, there may be significant cost in establishing centralized billing and management functions, ancillary services, and physical plant. Some of these will be capital costs, whereas others will be reflected as operating expense.

Depending on whether accounts receivable assets are part of the transaction, the working capital of the new entity may need to be considered as a cost. *Working capital* refers to general operating costs of the practice(s) incurred prior to receipt of payment for services. The more practices that are added and the faster the entity grows, the bigger the working capital investment. Typically this investment is offset, however, by a partial or complete ownership position in the accounts receivable.

The growth factor is a vital but frequently overlooked cost item. Participants should factor in the magnitude of incremental working capital costs, as well as capital costs related to practice acquisition or expansion. As illustrated in the Midwest Medical Center case study (chapter 6), a successful "overperforming" integration program can appear to be "underperforming" from a financial standpoint due to working capital requirements.

Based on the identified structural relationship, growth assumptions, anticipated infrastructure needs, and acquisition costs, a five-year financial analysis (described in chapter 2) can be established and modified. This analysis should include multiple scenarios that reflect variation in key assumptions, particularly revenue and production. The task force (also described in chapter 2) can evaluate costs associated with each scenario, discuss the implications of various alternatives, and reach a consensus on expectations. This makes the establishment of physician compensation incentives much easier, including shared risk and reward for overall performance.

☐ Political Issues

Three political issues challenge hospital–physician integration strategies. The first stems from the rapid change that characterizes the health care environment. Health care delivery and financing systems are in transition—from fee-for-service, episodic care delivery to prospective capitated payment and management of costs and health outcomes for defined populations. The business structure and incentives designed for one system may be ill suited, even detrimental, to another. Implementing effective incentives and workable organizational structures is complicated under either system.

From a politics standpoint, hospitals must walk a tightrope between investment in primary care and, during the transition period, maintenance of good relationships with the rest of the medical staff. Primary care physicians ultimately constitute the strongest asset under managed care and capitation and almost always are the focus of hospital–physician integration efforts. However, in a fee-for-service environment, all physicians, particularly big admitters and surgeons, continue to be extremely important to the bottom line.

What that means is that hospitals invest heavily in integration efforts with physicians in targeted specialties (primary care) and create assistance programs for the rest of the medical staff. In addition, specialists benefit from an enhanced base of primary care physicians and usually see this as a means to ensure or improve the future security of their referral streams.

A second and related political issue is that to be effective, not all specialists in any one specialty will be desirable participants. As physicians and health care providers of all types scramble for a shrinking pie of referrals, the gains of some will be at the expense of others. Health care organizations will identify and invest in their highest priorities. In striving to be attractive to purchasers, they will maximize cost-effectiveness and attempt to demonstrate quality outcomes. Physicians will be evaluated against these priorities, and, consequently, some will be excluded.

The third issue is that two types of nonparticipant physicians should be considered in the hospital's integration efforts. The first group is composed of physicians who either are not in demand or not considered a priority. The second type includes physicians who do not want to participate in a highly integrated relationship. To accommodate the latter group, hospitals are developing a continuum of services, enabling physicians to participate in an integrated relationship over time and at a level with which they are comfortable. However, this can foster an unwieldy management situation, resulting in a hodge-podge of business relationships between hospital and physicians. This business approach should be encouraged only for a specified period during transition, and physicians should be made to understand the organization's ultimate vision so as to prompt their movement toward more integration over time. However, physicians are likely to be willing to do this only to the extent that they are comfortable with the performance of the integrated entity and confident of the entity's chance for success in the market.

☐ Control and Decision Making

No party to an integration strategy wants to give up control, but full control can be maintained only through autonomy, and autonomous entities are at a competitive disadvantage and may risk obsolescence. This reality is the catalyst for discussing integration in the first place. Even so, cultural idiosyncracies and past organizational and operational patterns of the respective parties significantly affect the way individuals operate in the future. Neither party will find it easy to change a mind-set fixed by past experience. The educational and relationship-building process explained in chapter 2 is the starting point for this change in thought and behavior.

Formal ownership does not necessarily mean control, nor need it automatically result in the owner bearing full impact of the entity's financial performance. Control and responsibility for decision making should be evaluated carefully and allocated appropriately during the negotiation process. Instead of safeguarding the status quo, parties should structure decision-making systems so that the organization has the best possible foundation for effecting change and repositioning itself for managed care.

Because the term *control* evokes different responses in negotiating parties, they must separate the various categories of issues to be resolved. Only then can they identify their respective positions.

Integration activity in California prompted the California Medical Association (CMA) to analyze the implications that proposed ventures may have for their constituents' professional autonomy. After a great deal of deliberation, the CMA recently developed a document entitled *Decision-Making Authority for Integrated Entities Criteria*, listing the major areas of interest to physicians contemplating participation in an integrated entity. The result was delineation of decision-making authority among the "appropriate" decision maker, physician group, lay entity, or some level of collaboration between the two, based on the need to protect professional medical judgment. (See figure 4-6.)

This research is useful in two ways. First, it itemizes key issues that arise for decision-making authority in an integrated entity. Second, it provides a model, or a starting point, for the sensitive discussion of control and decision making for negotiating entities.

Once authorities have been identified for the collaborative entity, consideration must be given to the mechanics of decision making. This often depends on the size of the group, the frequency and complexity of issues requiring high-level decision making, and the parties' prior experience with this type of decision making. As a rule, decision-making levels include the board, subcommittees with appointed or elected representation, and designated leaders (typically paid positions). Task forces may be appointed to deal with specific issues that are temporary or intermittent. As demonstrated in the CMA model, the three far-left columns and the three far-right columns could be addressed by medical leaders and lay leaders respectively. However, decisions requiring formal consultation, consensus, or recommendations would likely be handled by the board or a committee. Board subcommittees could be formed based on the level and quantity of issues that require formal discussion or recommendations.

☐ Leadership

Regardless of what structure and decision-making controls are established at the outset, conflicts are inevitable and require strong and savvy leadership. Some affiliations may provide for co-equal leadership between physicians and nonphysicians. Their working relationship with one another and with their respective constituencies is crucial. Furthermore, mutual respect must be ensured between lay participant/owners and medical participant/owners.

There is general understanding of the role of the lay administrator/leader. On the other hand, the role of the physician leader—the *medical director*—is rapidly evolving into

Figure 4-6. Decision-Making Authority for Integrated Entities

Practicing Physicians Make Ultimate Decision			Neither Party May Solely Make Ultimate Decision	Lay Entity Makes Ultimate Decision		
No Duty to Consult / *Exclusive*	Informal Advice / *Consultative*	Formal Recommendation / *Shared*	Formal Consultation and Agreement / *Joint*	Formal Recommendation / *Shared*	Informal Advice / *Consultative*	No Duty to Consult / *Exclusive*
• Setting purely medical practice policies • What conditions can be referred to another physician specialist • What diagnostic tests are appropriate for a particular condition • What gets included in a particular patient's medical records • Whether a particular patient visit requires a particular billing code • Communications with patients of a purely clinical nature • Determination as to whether an emergency exists	• Practice parameters • Making treatment decisions that involve biomedical ethics • Credentialing for specific procedures: establishing general standards and as applied to individuals • Scheduling on-call coverage • Handling impaired physicians • Which CME courses should be taken • Terminating physicians from practice arrangements on discretionary grounds, that is, quality-of-care and business concerns, failure to comply with UR procedures, "without cause"	• Allocating resources • Establishing bioethics policies • Types of technology, new or old, which should be employed • To whom a physician can refer • Credentialing—establishing the standards for admission to the group[1] • Credentialing—an individual application for admission to the group[1] • Developing a UR and QA plan[1] • Implementing a UR and QA plan • Enforcing the UR and QA plan (except terminations from groups) • Whether and when to utilize limited license practitioners[1] • Determining whether to consider an application for admission • Selecting independent LLPs and "physician extenders" • Developing drug formularies • Selecting key administrative—medical officers[1] • How many patients a physician should see[1] • Controlling medical data • Terminating physicians from practice arrangements on nondiscretionary grounds[2]	• How many hours a physician should work • Nonclinical decisions concerning medical records • Contractual relationships with third-party payers • Level and scope of malpractice coverage • How much the physician group (including cost of all benefits) should be compensated • Setting cases for all parties named • Marketing • Setting the global budget for limited-license practitioner compensation • Establishing grievance policies • Making a decision to transfer a patient • Mergers, acquisitions, conversions, and affiliations[3] • Ownership and scope of ancillary ventures[3] • Level of indigent care provided • Employment matters • How much the lay entity, including the entity's executive management, should be compensated	• Selecting non-physician-dependent practitioners only • Selecting key administrative positions • Purchasing, replacing, and repairing equipment • How much patients should pay[1]	• Coding and billing procedures • Controlling administrative data	• Compensation for allied health and lay staff • Selecting purely administrative staff that do not hold key positions

[1] In these "shared" decisions, approval of the recommendations must not be withheld absent convincing justification transmitted in writing.

[2] Nondiscretionary grounds can be loss of licensure, Medicare/Medi-Cal exclusion, precredentialing mistakes, lack of board certification, and lack of or insufficient liability insurance.

[3] These decisions may ultimately rest with either party, depending on the nature of the relationship between the physician group and lay entity.

Note: An integrated entity is defined as an entity where there has been a consolidation of practicing physicians and lay business(es) into a health delivery system(s). Excluded from this definition are (1) the traditional organized hospital medical staff and (2) entities licensed under the Knox–Keene Act, which are exempted by virtue of the Act's regulatory scheme. Additionally, authority can be defined in the following ways:

| MD | | LE | Exclusive: | Physician (MD) or lay entity (LE) has sole responsibility for the decision. Neither party has a duty to consult with the other, even on an informal basis. |

MD → LE
MD → LE   Consultive: Physician or lay entity is encouraged to informally seek or receive information or advice from the other, but each retains ultimate decision-making authority.

MD [↑] LE   Shared: As a prerequisite to final action, the physician or lay entity makes a recommendation to the other through a formal process. Although the ultimate decision-making authority rests with the party receiving the recommendation, the recommendation, in light of the significance of the interest involved, is entitled to careful consideration.

MD [↓] LE   Shared:[1] Although the ultimate decision-making authority still rests with the party receiving the recommendation, the legitimate interests of the party making the recommendation require that adoption of the recommendation not be withheld absent convincing justification transmitted in writing.

| MD/LE | Joint: | Both the physician and the lay entity must agree when making a decision. |

Source: ©California Medical Association, 1994. Published with permission of and by arrangement with the California Medical Association. Copies of the preceding criteria, as well as an accompanying white paper entitled "The Corporate Practice of Medicine Bar—A Framework for Compliance," may be obtained from the California Medical Association by calling (415) 882-5144.

a key position of responsibility in an integrated delivery system, as shown by the profile in figure 4-7.

Candidates for this role may already be apparent at the beginning of the integration process. Some of the best candidates emerge from integration discussions—individuals known and trusted by their peers—and their leadership and potential contribution likely has become apparent to other participants in the planning process. Another option is to recruit a physician leader from the outside, perhaps through a search firm.

Once a medical director is selected, organizational support in terms of resources and continuing education must be extended to this person so that he or she can stay abreast of changing developments in health care nationally, regionally, and locally. In this way, the individual not only adds value as a visionary and strategic thinker, but he or she also is able to help the various participants, physicians in particular, maintain a balanced perspective on the alternatives to change.

□ Conclusion

The business issues outlined in this chapter are fairly generic, common to each affiliation situation. However, the most difficult business issues often are circumstantial and therefore unique to each situation. The case studies in part two offer practical insight as to how various organizations have dealt with these unique circumstances.

Figure 4-7. Medical Director Profile/Job Description

Physician Leadership

- Set and articulate vision.
- Gain physician commitment and support.
- Lead physicians through transition issues.
- Mediate physician conflicts.

Planning

- Assist with mission statement and overall goals.
- Determine clinical program needs.
- Plan physician recruiting.
- Establish financial targets based on medical costs.
- Review third-party contracts.

Managed Care Functions

- Develop managed care network.
- Assess reimbursement rates.
- Promote preventive medicine.
- Monitor managed care performance.

Clinical Oversight

- Develop and implement medical policy.
- Advocate physician performance review—QA, UR, and so forth.
- Coordinate education programs.
- Evaluate physician support roles.

Administration

- Market clinical programs.
- Coordinate physician income distribution arrangement.
- Provide input on information systems needs.
- Develop budgets.
- Respond to patient care problems.
- Act as a liaison between physicians and administration.

Source: Adapted from *Integrated Healthcare Report*, July 1993.

References

1. Kaiser, C. F., and Reilly, J. F. *Continuing Professional Education Exempt Organizations Technical Instruction Program for FY 1994.* Washington, DC: U.S. Government Printing Office, 1993, p. 235.

2. Kaiser and Reilly, pp. 235–36.

3. Cimasi, R. J. Valuing medical practices. In: T. L. West and J. D. Jones, editors. *Handbook of Business Valuation.* New York City: John Wiley & Sons, 1992, p. 274.

4. Revenue Ruling 68-609, 1968-2, C.B. 327.

5. Revenue Ruling 76-91, 1976-1, C.B. 149.

6. Grant, P. N. IRS approves exemption for medical group practices in integrated delivery system. *Journal of Taxation of Exempt Organizations,* July/Aug. 1993, p. 7.

7. Grant, p. 7.

Bibliography

Grant, P. N. IRS approves exemption for medical group practices in integrated delivery system. *Journal of Taxation of Exempt Organizations,* July/Aug. 1993, p. 3–7.

Jackson, J. B., and Hill, R. K. *New Trends in Dental Practice Valuation and Associateship Arrangements.* Chicago: Quintessence, 1987.

Kaiser, C. F., and Reilly, J. F. Integrated delivery systems. In: C. F. Kaiser and J. F. Reilly. *Continuing Professional Education Exempt Organizations Technical Instruction Program for FY 1994.* Washington, DC: U.S. Government Printing Office, 1993.

Pratt, S. P. *Valuing Small Businesses and Professional Practices.* 2nd ed. Homewood, IL: Business One Irwin, 1993.

West, T. L., and Jones, J. D., editors. *Handbook of Business Valuation.* New York City: John Wiley & Sons, 1992.

Chapter 5

Legal Issues

Thomas J. Onusko, Esq.

At the very time that hospitals and physicians are being driven by changes in the health care marketplace to seek closer relationships with each other, such relationships are being subjected to even closer legal scrutiny by courts and regulators. It is even more frustrating than it is ironic that federal and state governments, which encourage the formation of hospital–physician integrated delivery systems as a method of reducing health care costs, at the same time are fueling the legal risks that arise from such relationships.

The challenge for hospitals and physician group practices seeking to affiliate with each other in today's legal environment is to carefully examine the business goals of the proposed relationship and the legal issues they present. This examination will require consultation with experienced legal counsel to design an organizational structure that comes closest to achieving the desired business goals while at the same time minimizing inherent legal risks.

This chapter will address six major legal issues surrounding integrative relationships:

1. Fraud and abuse (investment, space and equipment rental, personal service and management contracts, sale of practice, employees, managed care plans)
2. Physician self-referrals (the Stark Bill and certain exceptions including physician services, in-office ancillary services, prepaid plans, and ownership in publicly held entities)
3. Tax-exempt status (private inurement, with special emphasis on purchasing group practice assets and compensation; qualifying for tax-exempt status)
4. Corporate practice of medicine (fee-splitting sanctions and penalties, physician employment and compensation, strategies for avoiding violation)
5. Antitrust regulation (safeguards against Sherman Act violation and penalties, antitrust "safety zones")
6. Employee benefit plans (qualified and nonqualified plans, qualification tests, controlled group rules, and so forth)

The issues covered in this chapter are by no means exhaustive. However, upon reading the material provided here affiliation planners and involved parties – under full guidance of expert legal counsel – will have a good sense of the key legal implications of their negotiation process.

☐ Fraud and Abuse

The federal antikickback statute prohibits the knowing and willful payment or receipt of any direct or indirect remuneration in return for referring, arranging, or recommending the referral of a patient, or purchasing, leasing, ordering, or arranging for any good, facility, service, or item to be paid by either the Medicare or Medicaid program.[1] Violators are subject to criminal penalties and/or civil remedies, including exclusion from the Medicare and Medicaid programs; fines of up to $25,000 per violation; and imprisonment for up to five years.

Many states have adopted their own version of the federal antikickback statute.[2] These state statutes are even broader in their application than the federal statute, because typically state laws are not limited to referrals of Medicare and Medicaid items and services but prohibit remuneration for *any* type of referral.

This broad proscription against remuneration in return for referrals is applied using the very subjective "one-purpose" test adopted by the federal courts.[3] Under this test, any form of remuneration paid by any person or entity receiving a referral to the person or entity making or arranging for such referral is illegal if even one purpose of the remuneration is to induce such referral, even if there are other legitimate purposes for the remuneration. In other words, the inducement to refer does not have to be the primary purpose of the remuneration; so long as it is even one purpose, the remuneration is illegal under the federal statute.

Congress recognized that the federal antikickback statute is written so broadly and applied so subjectively that it would prohibit many relatively innocuous or even beneficial commercial arrangements between health care providers. Therefore, in 1987 Congress required the Office of Inspector General (OIG) to promulgate regulations specifying which payment practices will *not* be subject to criminal prosecution and/or civil remedies. Unfortunately, these "safe harbors" are drafted so narrowly that they do not protect many relatively common and otherwise legitimate types of provider transactions.

In light of the foregoing, any transaction involving remuneration between a hospital and physician(s) presents inherent fraud and abuse risks, where either party is the source of referrals for the other. In the context of a hospital affiliation with a group practice that is a referral source for the hospital, or vice versa, significant fraud and abuse issues are presented. The only way to avoid risk is to qualify the various aspects of the transaction under an appropriate safe harbor.

Failure to satisfy safe-harbor requirements does not necessarily mean a transaction is illegal. It merely means that the transaction is subject to scrutiny under the one-purpose test. As a practical matter, the more safe-harbor requirements a transaction satisfies, the less likely an investigation and/or prosecution will result. Following are descriptions of areas treated within the safe harbors.

Investment Interests

There are two *existing* and three *proposed* safe harbors for investment interests. The two existing ones are for publicly held entities and for small entities that satisfy the two so-called 60–40 tests. The three proposed safe harbors are for small entities located in rural areas, ambulatory surgical centers, and group practices. Although the two existing investment interest safe harbors afford little protection for hospital affiliations with physician group practices, the three proposed investment interest safe harbors may provide protection for at least certain aspects of such an affiliation, depending on the circumstances.

There is an existing safe harbor for investment interests in *public corporations*, that is, those that have more than $50 million in undepreciated net tangible assets. Unless the proposed affiliation will involve a national hospital chain having assets in such magnitude, this safe harbor offers no protection for a hospital–physician group affiliation.

The other existing safe harbor protects investment interests in small entities that satisfy certain criteria. The most important of these criteria are the two so-called 60–40 tests, that is, that not more than 40 percent of the entity's ownership can be held (ownership test) and not more than 40 percent of the entity's revenues can be generated (revenue test) by persons or entities in a position to make or influence referrals to, furnish items or services to, or otherwise generate business for the entity. Because both the hospital and the physician group will either be making referrals to, furnishing items or services to, or otherwise generating business for any entity resulting from an affiliation between them, such entity would not satisfy the 60–40 ownership test and probably would not satisfy the 60–40 revenue test. However, there are three new proposed safe harbors for investment interests in small entities that do not require compliance with either of the 60–40 tests.

Small Entities Located in Rural Areas
There is a proposed safe harbor for investment interests in small entities located in rural areas, that is, areas outside a standard metropolitan statistical area (SMSA). Because the OIG recognizes that physicians are often the only source of capital in such areas, and because physicians located in such areas often do not have alternate facilities to which they can refer, the OIG has proposed a safe harbor that protects this category of investments so long as the following eight criteria are satisfied:

1. An equal and bona fide opportunity to acquire investment interests in the entity must be offered to persons or entities irrespective of their ability to make or influence referrals to, provide items or services to, or generate business for the entity.
2. The terms on which an investment interest is offered to a passive investor who is in a position to make or influence referrals to, furnish items or services to, or generate business for the entity must be no different from the terms offered to other passive investors.
3. The terms on which an investment interest is offered cannot be related to previous or expected volume of referrals, items or services furnished, or the amount of business otherwise generated from the investor to the entity.
4. There can be no requirement that a passive investor make referrals to, provide items or services to, or otherwise generate business for the entity as a condition for remaining an investor.
5. The entity or any investor must not market or furnish the entity's items or services to passive investors any differently than is the case for noninvestors.
6. At least 85 percent of the dollar volume of the entity's business in the previous fiscal year or previous 12-month period must be derived from the service of persons who reside in a rural area.
7. The entity or any investor must not make or guarantee loans to any investor in a position to make or influence referrals to, provide items or services to, or otherwise generate business for the entity if the investor uses any part of such loan to obtain the investment interest.
8. The return to an investor must be directly proportional to the amount of the capital investment of that investor.

This proposed safe harbor would permit the formation of a jointly owned hospital-physician group entity so long as the entity was located in and primarily served a "rural" area and satisfied the other criteria of the proposed safe harbor.

Medicare-Certified Ambulatory Surgery Centers
A second proposed safe harbor would permit investment interests in Medicare-certified ambulatory surgical centers where all the investors are surgeons who refer patients directly to such center and perform the surgeries on the referred patients. This proposal contains the following five standards:

1. No investor can be offered better investment terms based on past or expected referrals or amounts of services furnished to the entity.
2. A passive investor may not be required to make referrals to the entity in order to continue as an investor.
3. Neither the entity nor any investor may loan funds or guarantee funds to an investor for use in obtaining an investment interest.
4. Payments may not be made based on the level of referrals.
5. The investor surgeon must agree to treat Medicare and Medicaid patients.

Unfortunately, as currently proposed this safe harbor would not protect a hospital investment in an ambulatory surgical center along with the surgeons. However, in the comments to the proposed safe harbor, the OIG has indicated that it is considering expanding the scope of this proposed safe harbor to protect other types of investors as well. If the hospital would be a truly passive investor in an ambulatory surgical center joint venture (that is, would not make referrals to, provide items or services to, or otherwise arrange business for the center) with a group of surgeons, the fraud and abuse risk may be reduced, even if the transaction would not qualify under the proposed safe harbor.

Group Practices Composed Exclusively of Active Investors
The third proposed safe harbor in this area would protect investment interests in group practices composed exclusively of active investors. For purposes of this safe harbor, *active investor* is defined to include only investors who are either responsible for the day-to-day management of the entity and are bona fide general partners in a partnership, or who agree in writing to undertake liability for the actions of the entity's agents acting within the scope of their agency. To qualify as a "group practice" investors must satisfy the following three standards:

1. Physician members of the group provide substantially the full range of their services through the shared use of office space, facilities, equipment, and personnel.
2. Substantially all services of the members are provided through the group and billed through the group, with payments received as receipts of the group.
3. Overhead expenses and income of the group are distributed in accordance with a predetermined formula.

As currently proposed, the safe harbor would only protect physicians who form themselves into a group practice. However, the OIG has indicated that it is considering expanding the scope of this proposed safe harbor to protect other types of investors, including hospitals and passive investors who are not in a position to make referrals.

Space and Equipment Rental

These existing safe harbors protect space and equipment rental, so long as the lease meets the following five criteria:

1. The lease is in writing and signed by the parties.
2. Lease terms specify precisely what premises and/or equipment is being leased.
3. Lease terms specify the exact periods of usage and rental.
4. The lease is for a term of at least one year.
5. Lease terms provide for a rent that is set in advance and consistent with fair market value and does not take into account the volume or value of any referrals.

These safe harbors would protect any lease arrangement between a hospital and a physician group so long as these five criteria are satisfied. It is important to note that in light of the fifth criterion, some revenue leases are not protected.

Personal Service and Management Contracts

This existing safe harbor protects payments made by a principal to an agent as compensation for personal or management services rendered by the agent, so long as the agreement meets the following six criteria:

1. The contract is in writing and signed by the parties.
2. Terms of the contract specify the services to be provided.
3. If not a full-time arrangement, terms specify the exact schedule and duration of, as well as the exact charge for, such services.
4. The contract is for a term of at least one year.
5. The contract terms provide for aggregate compensation that is set in advance, is consistent with fair market value, and does not take into account the volume or value of any referrals.
6. The services performed do not involve counseling with regard to, or performance of, an illegal activity.

Pursuant to this safe harbor, a hospital and a physician group could enter into a personal service or management contract whereby one party provides services for a fee to the other. It is important to note that because of the fifth criterion, the providing party cannot be compensated on a percentage-of-revenue, per-hour, or per-procedure basis and still qualify under this safe harbor.

Sale of Practice

As currently written, the safe harbor in this area only protects the sale of a practice by one practitioner to another where the sale is completed within one year and where after one year the seller will no longer be in a position to make referrals to the buyer. In its comments to the current safe harbor, the OIG criticizes hospital acquisitions of physician practices as a potentially abusive method for locking in referrals to the hospital. The OIG cites the example of a hospital acquiring a physician practice for an amount substantially in excess of the fair market value of the practice as deemed by another physician, which infers that the hospital is purchasing not just the value of the practice itself but the value of the referrals that flow to the hospital from the practice.

In a December 22, 1992, letter to the Internal Revenue Service, the associate general counsel of the OIG questioned the legality of a hospital's purchase of the intangible assets of a physician practice (that is, goodwill, noncompete agreement, patient records, and so forth). This purchase was within the context of the selling physician continuing to work for the practice after the sale.

In its comments to the proposed safe harbors, the OIG has invited comment as to whether safe-harbor protection should be extended to transactions involving the purchase by a rural hospital of a practice as part of a physician recruitment program, where the rural hospital buys and holds the practice of a retiring physician and employs locum tenens (stand-in or temporary) physicians to operate the practice until a new physician can be recruited to take over the practice. Although the acquisition of a group practice by a hospital is not currently protected by a safe harbor, if the hospital only purchases the tangible assets of the practice for their fair market value and does not pay for the value of the referrals from that practice to the hospital, the risk of a fraud and abuse violation is significantly reduced.

Employees

There is a statutory exception to the federal antikickback statute that protects payments by an employer to a bona fide employee for employment in the provision of covered items or services.[4] The existing safe harbor in this area protects compensation paid to persons who qualify as "employees" for purposes of the 1986 Internal Revenue Code, as amended (the Code). Where a hospital employs physicians in a group practice, compensation paid by the hospital to the physician employees for professional services rendered should be immune from fraud and abuse risk. However, the OIG has indicated that in its view, because the statutory exception only protects payments for "covered services," payments by an employer to a physician employee that represent a kickback of revenues generated by referrals by the physician employee for ancillary services are still illegal, despite the existence of an employment relationship.

Managed Care Plans

This safe harbor protects incentives offered by a health plan to an enrollee, as well as price reductions offered by a provider to a health plan, so long as certain criteria are satisfied. Unfortunately, this safe harbor only protects health plans that have Medicare contracts or are regulated under state laws relating to insurance companies, health maintenance organizations (HMOs), or preferred provider organizations (PPOs). Where a hospital forms a joint entity with a group practice to serve as a contracting vehicle with managed care plans, safe-harbor protection is not available unless the joint entity has a Medicare contract or is a state-regulated insurance company, HMO, or PPO. However, even if such a joint entity does not qualify as a "health plan" for purposes of the safe harbor, fraud and abuse risk at least can be reduced by complying with the other safe-harbor criteria.

With respect to incentives offered to enrollees, this basically means that the same incentives must be offered to Medicare and Medicaid enrollees as are offered to other types of enrollees, and that the health plan cannot seek to recover from Medicare or Medicaid the cost of any such incentive. With respect to health plan price reductions offered by providers, this basically means that there must be a written agreement between the provider and the health plan and that the health plan must report and pass the benefit of any discount through to the Medicare and Medicaid programs.

☐ Physician Self-Referrals

The Ethics in Patient Referrals Act of 1989 (the Stark Bill), as amended by the Omnibus Budget Reconciliation Act of 1993 (OBRA '93), prohibits a physician (or an immediate family member of a physician) who has a financial relationship with an entity from making a referral to the entity for the furnishing of a designated health service for which payment may be made under either the Medicare or Medicaid program.[5] The Stark Bill also prohibits such an entity from presenting a claim for payment to any individual or third-party payer for a designated health service furnished pursuant to a prohibited referral.

There are several penalties for violation of the Stark Bill. Medicare and Medicaid reimbursement is denied for a service that is provided pursuant to a prohibited referral. Any amount billed and collected from Medicare or Medicaid for a prohibited referral must be refunded. Any person presenting a bill or claim to Medicare or Medicaid for a service related to a prohibited referral is subject to a civil monetary penalty of not more than $15,000 per service. A physician or other entity that enters into an arrangement or scheme to circumvent prohibitions of the Stark Bill is subject to a civil monetary penalty of not more than $100,000. A violation of the bill may also be grounds for exclusion from the Medicare and Medicaid programs. Many states have adopted their own version of the bill and prohibit self-referrals by physicians for items or services reimbursable by *any* payer, not just Medicare or Medicaid.

The original version of the bill only prohibited self-referrals by physicians for clinical laboratory services. However, amendments in OBRA '93 expanded the scope of the statute (effective January 1, 1995) to prohibit self-referrals by physicians for *designated health services*, which are defined to include not only clinical laboratory services but also the following items:

- Physical and occupational therapy services
- Radiology or other diagnostic services
- Radiation therapy services
- Durable medical equipment
- Parenteral and enteral nutrients, equipment, and supplies
- Prosthetics, orthotics, and prosthetic devices
- Home health services
- Outpatient prescription drugs
- Inpatient and outpatient hospital services

The Stark Bill defines the term *financial relationship* to include both ownership and investment interests as well as compensation arrangements.

If a hospital–physician group affiliation will result in any type of physician ownership or investment interest in, or compensation arrangement with, the hospital or an affiliated entity to which the physicians will make referrals for designated health services, such an affiliation will violate the Stark Bill unless it satisfies one or more of the statutory exceptions contained therein. Several exceptions are contained in the bill that would protect various types of hospital–physician group affiliations. These exceptions are described in the following subsections.

Physician Services

This exception permits referrals to a physician in the same group practice as the referring physician. The term *group practice* means a group of two or more physicians organized legally as a partnership, professional corporation, foundation, not-for-profit corporation, faculty practice plan, or similar association that meets the following five criteria:

1. Each physician member of the group provides substantially the full range of services that the physician routinely provides through the joint use of shared office space, facilities, equipment, and personnel.
2. Substantially all services of the physician members of the group are provided through the group and are billed under a billing number assigned to the group, and amounts received are treated as receipts of the group.
3. Overhead expenses of, and income from, the practice are distributed in accordance with methods previously determined.
4. Except for permitted profit and productivity bonuses, no physician member of the group directly or indirectly receives compensation that is based on the volume or value of referrals by the physician.
5. Members of the group personally conduct not less than 75 percent of the physician–patient encounters of the group practice.

A physician in a group practice may be paid in a share of overall profits of the group, or a productivity bonus based on services personally performed or services incident to such personally performed services, so long as the share or bonus is not determined in a manner that is directly related to the volume or value of referrals by such physician.

In-Office Ancillary Services

This exception permits a referral by a physician for in-office ancillary services (other than durable medical equipment excluding infusion pumps and parenteral and enteral nutrients, equipment, and supplies), so long as the following conditions are met:

- Such services are furnished personally by the referring physician, by another physician member of the same group practice, or by individuals directly supervised by the referring physician or another physician in the same group practice.
- Such services are furnished in a building in which the referring physician (or another physician member of the same group practice) furnishes physician services unrelated to the furnishing of designated health services; or, in the case of a referring physician who is a member of a group practice, in another building that is used by the group practice for the provision of some or all of the group's clinical laboratory services or for the centralized provision of the group's designated health services (other than clinical laboratory services) that are billed by the physician performing or supervising the services, by a group practice of which such physician is a member under a billing number assigned to the group practice, or by an entity that is wholly owned by such physician or such group practice.

Prepaid Plans

This exception permits referrals by a physician to certain types of prepaid plans with which the physician has a financial relationship, including a qualified HMO. This exception, then, would permit a hospital–physician group affiliation that results in the formation of an HMO.

Ownership in Publicly Traded Securities and Mutual Funds

This exception protects physician referrals to certain types of publicly held entities in which a physician has an ownership or investment interest, including securities listed on a national or regional stock exchange in corporations that have stockholder equity exceeding $75 million. Where the hospital is owned by a national chain whose stock meets the definition of a *publicly held security,* this exception may protect an affiliation arrangement whereby the physician group acquires an ownership or investment interest in such corporation.

Rural Providers

This exception permits physician referrals to a rural provider in which the physician has an ownership or investment interest, if substantially all of the designated health services furnished by such entity are furnished to individuals who reside in such rural area. For purposes of this exception, the term *rural* is defined the same as in the proposed fraud and abuse safe harbors as described earlier, that is, geographic areas located outside an SMSA.

Hospital Ownership

This exception permits physician referrals to a hospital in which the physician has an ownership or investment interest. However, two conditions apply: (1) the referring physician is authorized to perform services at the hospital, and (2) the ownership or investment interest is in the hospital itself and not merely in a department of the hospital.

Rental of Office Space and Equipment

This exception permits physician referrals in an entity with which the physician has a compensation arrangement involving an office or equipment rental, so long as the following five criteria are met:

1. The lease is in writing, signed by the parties, and specifies the premises or equipment covered by the lease.
2. The space or equipment rented or leased does not exceed that which is reasonable and necessary for the legitimate business purposes of the lease or rental and is used exclusively by the lessee (except for common areas) when being used by the lessee.
3. The lease provides for a term of at least one year.
4. The rental charges over the term of the lease are set in advance, are consistent with fair market value, and are not determined in a manner that takes into account the volume or value of any referrals of other business generated between the parties.
5. The lease would be commercially reasonable even if no referrals were made between the parties.

Bona Fide Employment Relationships

This exception protects payments by an employer to a physician (or an immediate family member of such physician) who is a bona fide employee for the provision of services, if the following three criteria are met:

1. The employment is for identifiable services.
2. The amount of remuneration is consistent with the fair market value of the services and, except for productivity bonuses based on services performed personally by the physician (or an immediate family member of such physician), is not determined in a manner that takes into account (directly or indirectly) the volume or value of any referrals by the physician.
3. The remuneration is provided pursuant to an agreement that would be commercially reasonable even if no referrals were made to the employer.

Personal Service Contracts

This exception permits remuneration pursuant to a personal service contract with a physician, if the following six criteria are met:

1. The arrangement is set out in writing, signed by the parties, and specifies the services covered.
2. The arrangement covers all of the services to be provided by the physician (or an immediate family member of such physician).
3. The aggregate services contracted for do not exceed those that are reasonable and necessary for the legitimate business purposes of the arrangement.
4. The term of the arrangement is for at least one year.
5. The compensation to be paid over the term of the arrangement is set in advance; does not exceed fair market value; and, except in the case of a physician incentive plan, is not determined in a manner that takes into account the volume or value of any referrals or other business generated between the parties.
6. The services to be performed do not involve the counseling or promotion of a business arrangement or other activity that violates any state or federal law.

In contrast to the similar fraud and abuse safe harbor for personal service contracts, it is important to note that the fifth criterion for the Stark exception for personal service contracts does not require that the "aggregate" amount of compensation be set in advance. Thus, although a per-hour or per-procedure compensation arrangement would not qualify for protection under the fraud and abuse safe harbor, it would be protected under the Stark exception, so long as the other criteria were satisfied. A percentage-of-revenue compensation arrangement, however, would be problematic for both fraud and abuse and Stark purposes.

In the case of physician incentive plans, compensation may be determined in a manner (a withhold, capitation, bonus, or otherwise) that takes into account directly or indirectly the volume or value of any referrals or other business generated between the parties, if the plan meets the following three requirements:

1. No specific payment is made directly or indirectly under the plan to a physician or a physician group as an inducement to reduce or limit medically necessary services.
2. In the case of a plan that places a physician or physician group at substantial financial risk, the plan complies with any requirements the secretary of the Department of Health and Human Services may impose.
3. Upon request by the secretary, the entity provides the secretary with access to descriptive information regarding the plan in order to permit the secretary to determine whether the plan is in compliance with the requirements of this exception.

The term *physician incentive plan* means any compensation arrangement between an entity and a physician or physician group that may directly or indirectly have the effect of reducing or limiting services provided with respect to individuals enrolled with the entity.

Remuneration Unrelated to the Provision of Designated Health Services

This exception permits a hospital to pay remuneration to a physician if such remuneration is not related to the provision of designated health services. For example, a hospital would be protected by this exception if it paid a physician to provide administrative services, such as serving as the hospital's quality assurance director or as a department chair, so long as the compensation did not relate to the providing of a designated health service by such physician.

Isolated Transactions

This exception permits isolated financial transactions between a hospital and a physician group practice, such as a one-time sale of property or practice, if the following two conditions are met:

1. The amount of remuneration paid is consistent with the fair market value of the item or items being sold and not determined in a manner that takes into account (directly or indirectly) the volume or value of any referrals by the physicians.
2. The remuneration is provided pursuant to an agreement that would be commercially reasonable even if no referrals were made to the purchaser.

Group Practice Arrangements with a Hospital

This exception permits an arrangement between a hospital and a physician group under which designated health services are provided by the group but billed by the hospital, if the following six criteria are met:

1. With respect to the services provided to an inpatient of the hospital, the services are diagnostic or therapeutic items or services ordinarily furnished to inpatients by the hospital or by others under arrangements with the hospital.
2. The arrangement began prior to December 19, 1989, and has continued in effect without interruption since such date.

3. With respect to the designated health services covered under the arrangement, substantially all such services furnished to patients of the hospital are furnished by the group under the arrangement.
4. The arrangement is pursuant to an agreement that is set out in writing and specifies the services to be provided by the parties and the compensation for services provided under the agreement.
5. The compensation paid over the term of the agreement is consistent with fair market value, and the compensation per unit of service is fixed in advance and is not determined in a manner that takes into account the volume or value of referrals or other business generated between the parties.
6. The compensation is provided pursuant to an agreement that would be commercially reasonable even if no referrals were made to the entity.

Payments by a Physician for Items and Services

This exception protects payments made by a physician to a laboratory in exchange for the provision of clinical laboratory services, or to an entity as compensation for other items or services if the items or services are furnished at a price that is consistent with fair market value. Absent this exception, the providing of items or services to a physician by an entity would constitute a form of remuneration, such that if the physician made referrals to the entity, the physician would be deemed to have a compensation arrangement with the entity in violation of the Stark Bill.

Proposed Changes to Stark Exceptions

Several of the health care reform proposals pending in Congress as of this writing, including President Clinton's Health Security Act, would significantly modify the Stark exceptions described in the preceding sections in an effort to fight health care fraud. In addition to increasing the investigatory powers of enforcement entities and the penalties for a violation of either the fraud and abuse or the self-referral statute, the exceptions to the Stark Bill described in the preceding sections would be narrowed, making it even more difficult for hospitals and physicians to undertake alliances. The proposed changes to the Stark Bill exceptions include the following:

- Repealing the existing exception for physician services provided personally by or under the supervision of another physician in the same group practice as the referring physician
- Limiting the in-office ancillary service exceptions to clinical lab, X-ray, and ultrasound services that are provided at low cost
- Limiting the existing exception for prepaid plans while adding a new general exception for capitated plans
- Modifying the rural provider exception to require at least 85 percent (rather than "substantially all") of the designated health services to be furnished to persons residing in the rural area
- Repealing the exception for remuneration paid by a hospital to a physician if the remuneration does not relate to designated health services
- Limiting the physician recruitment exception to entities in rural areas or health professional shortage areas or to entities that receive community health center grants from the Public Health Service
- Making the isolated transaction exception unavailable if there is a financing between the parties, thus permitting only one-time payments for sales of property and practices by physicians to hospitals

Although the passage of President Clinton's Health Security Act, or any of the other health care reform proposals pending in Congress as of this writing, is facing increasing obstacles, it is very possible that some or all of the changes to the Stark exceptions could be passed by the Congress in the meantime. Representative Pete Stark introduced a separate bill in March 1994 containing the preceding changes, giving Congress the option of adopting the changes with or without a comprehensive piece of health care reform legislation.

☐ Tax-Exempt Status

Many hospitals and physician clinics throughout the country historically have been organized as tax-exempt organizations pursuant to Section 501(c)(3) of the Internal Revenue Code (IRC). Tax-exempt organizations enjoy many benefits, such as avoidance of many forms of taxation, including federal and state income taxation and local real property taxation; access to tax-exempt financing; and deductibility of donations.

In the context of a hospital–physician group affiliation, two tax exemption issues may arise. First, if the hospital and/or the physician group is a tax-exempt organization, how will the proposed affiliation affect the tax-exempt status? Second, if the combined entity resulting from the affiliation desires to obtain tax-exempt status, how must the transaction and the entity be structured so as to obtain and maintain tax-exempt status? These questions are addressed in the following sections.

Private Inurement

Section 501(c)(3) of the IRC provides tax-exempt status for organizations that are "organized and operated exclusively for religious, charitable, scientific . . . or educational purposes . . . no part of the net earnings of which inures to the benefit of any private shareholder or individual. . . ." The language ". . . no part of the net earnings of which inures to the benefit of any private shareholder or individual . . ." gives rise to the prohibition against private inurement.

In its simplest terms, the *private inurement test,* according to the IRS, "means that a private shareholder or individual cannot pocket the organization's funds except as reasonable payment for goods or services."[6] This prohibition against inurement applies to insiders of the organization. The IRS has determined that members of a hospital's medical staff who refer patients to the hospital are "insiders" for purposes of the private inurement rule.[7]

In recent years the IRS has scrutinized relationships between tax-exempt hospitals and physicians more closely to determine whether a financial transaction between them results in impermissible private inurement.[8] The purpose of the private inurement test is to make sure that insiders do not, by reason of their position, improperly acquire any funds of a tax-exempt organization. This is not to say that such persons may not receive reasonable compensation for goods or services provided to an exempt organization in conjunction with the furtherance of the exempt organization's exempt purposes. For example, employees of an exempt organization may be paid reasonable wages. Although there are numerous economic benefits to which the private inurement rule might apply, the receipt of an economic benefit by an insider gives rise to an inurement problem only if the exempt organization does not receive fair value in return. Private inurement does not include a compensation arrangement (even with a person considered to be an insider) if the amount of compensation paid the individual is reasonable relative to the goods or services provided by that individual to the exempt organization.

Two components of hospital–physician group affiliations present significant private inurement risks. The first involves any purchase price paid by a hospital to acquire assets of the physician group practice, and the second has to do with any compensation paid by a hospital to the physicians for their ongoing professional services.

Purchase of Group Practice Assets

A tax-exempt hospital must clearly articulate the charitable purpose being furthered by the proposed acquisition and why it is the least costly alternative for achieving that charitable purpose. Negotiations must be conducted on an arm's-length basis, and the purchase price for the assets should not exceed fair market value as supported by independent appraisals. As discussed previously in this chapter, if the hospital proposes to acquire intangible assets (such as goodwill) of a physician group practice that refers patients to the hospital, this can present significant fraud and abuse risks. A violation of the fraud and abuse laws also jeopardizes a hospital's tax-exempt status.[9] To avoid risk and the attendant private inurement issue, the hospital must take care to base the purchase price for the practice on the value of future referrals to the practice (that is, the value to another practitioner), rather than on the value of referrals from the practice to the hospital.

Compensation for Professional Services

With respect to compensation to be paid by the hospital to the physicians for professional services, such compensation should be reasonable in light of the fair market value of services actually rendered by the physicians. To avoid liability for fraud and abuse and the attendant private inurement risk, any such arrangement should satisfy the requirements of the personal service contract safe harbor as discussed earlier in this chapter, including the requirement that the aggregate amount of such compensation be fixed and not vary with the volume or value of physician referrals to the hospital.

Qualifying for Tax-Exempt Status

Three basic structural options are available with respect to the tax status of the entity that results from a hospital–physician group affiliation: taxable corporation, tax-exempt organization, or nonprofit corporation subject to federal income taxation. A *taxable corporation* would not have to satisfy any of the requirements of Section 501(c)(3) of the Code and would be free to distribute its net earnings to private shareholders such as the physicians. However, unless the corporation qualifies as a Subchapter S corporation, it will be subject to double taxation—that is, the income will be subject to taxation and any income distributions to physician shareholders will be taxed a second time. Because Subchapter S corporations cannot have corporate shareholders (such as hospital corporations), this is not an alternative for most hospital–group practice affiliations.

Qualifying the entity as a *tax-exempt organization* would avoid double taxation because the entity would pay no tax on its net earnings. Only the compensation paid to physicians by the entity would be taxable. However, qualifying such an entity for tax-exempt status has become increasingly difficult and would subject the entity to a number of limitations in terms of its organization and operation. Applying for tax-exempt status can be a time-consuming and expensive process.

A third alternative is to organize the entity as a *nonprofit corporation under state law and subject to federal income taxation*. Depending on the laws of a particular state, such nonprofit corporation may enjoy exemption from various state forms of taxation, even though its net earnings would be subject to federal income taxation.

Organizational and Operational Tests

If the parties desire to obtain tax-exempt status, the entity will have to demonstrate to the IRS that it meets both the organizational and operational tests. To satisfy the *organizational test*, the organization's governing documents must limit organizational activities to carrying on recognized exempt purposes, limit lobbying and political campaign activities that can be conducted by the organization, and dedicate organizational assets (even upon dissolution) to such exempt purposes. To meet the *operational test*, the organization must conduct activities that seek to accomplish its exempt purposes. Traditionally the IRS has applied a community benefit test for the purpose of determining whether an entity that provides health care services is entitled to tax-exempt status. This test, based largely on Revenue Ruling 69-545, provides that to have tax-exempt status a health care provider must promote the health of a population segment that is broad enough to benefit the community as evidenced by a number of indicators. These indicators include the following:

- Control of the entity by an independent board of trustees that is representative of the community
- Maintenance of an open medical staff
- Operation of an emergency room that is open to all without regard to their ability to pay
- Provision of health care services to all persons in the community who are able to pay
- Use of excess funds to further exempt purposes

In light of the foregoing criteria, it would be difficult but not impossible for a hospital–physician group affiliation entity to qualify for tax-exempt status. Hospital–physician joint ventures have been under close scrutiny by the IRS since issuance of General Counsel Memorandum 39862, in which the IRS expressed its disapproval of prior private letter rulings approving joint ventures that involve the purchase by private physicians of the revenue streams of various hospital departments. The ruling indicated that it was not sufficient for a hospital to justify such a transaction on a cost-benefit analysis based on the hospital's bottom line; instead, the transaction must be justified based on the benefit to the community from such a transaction. However, in 1993 the IRS issued two rulings (discussed in the following subsection) in which it granted tax-exempt status to integrated delivery systems formed by hospitals and physicians.

Friendly Hills and *Facey Foundation* Rulings

In the *Friendly Hills* ruling, a tax-exempt hospital created a nonprofit corporation of which the hospital was the sole corporate member. The board of the new corporation was to be controlled by community representatives, with no more than 20 percent of board positions held by physicians. The new nonprofit entity purchased the assets of a physician group, including real estate, a general acute care hospital, 10 clinic facilities, and certain intangible assets (including noncompete covenants, HMO contracts, warranty rights, and prepaid assets) for a total purchase price of $110 million, which was represented to be at or below the fair market value of the acquired assets. The new nonprofit corporation was to operate the hospital and clinic facilities purchased from the physician group, including operating an emergency room that was open to the public and provided care to all persons without regard to their ability to pay; conducting significant programs of medical research and health education; and participating in the Medicare and Medi-Cal programs. The new nonprofit corporation entered into a professional services agreement with a new professional corporation formed by the selling physicians pursuant to which the physicians were to be compensated on a capitated basis.

In the *Facey Foundation* ruling, the facts were similar in substance to the *Friendly Hills* case. A nonprofit corporation was formed as a subsidiary of a tax-exempt health care provider. Another taxable subsidiary of the parent purchased the stock of a physician group that operated five clinics. A portion of the stock's value was based on certain intangible assets (the group's trade name, patient files and records, software, a workforce in place, contracts to provide services, noncompete agreements, and goodwill). The new corporation was to lease or license from its taxable affiliate the assets acquired through the purchase of the group stock. It was represented to the IRS that all assets were to be acquired or leased at or below fair market value. The new corporation entered into a 20-year professional services agreement with a new professional corporation formed by selling physicians, which called for compensation for the first two years based on a percentage of adjusted gross revenue, 80 to 85 percent of which was to be derived from capitated contracts. Subsequent compensation was to be determined on the basis of arm's-length negotiation between the new professional corporation and the new nonprofit corporation, and it was represented to the IRS that the rates negotiated would reflect competitive rates for medical services and would not exceed reasonable compensation. The new corporation indicated that it would treat patients at its urgent care centers without regard to a patient's ability to pay, and the professional services agreement included a covenant that the physicians would not discriminate against individual patients based on ability to pay and would participate in both the Medicare and Medi-Cal programs without discrimination. The new corporation also intended to conduct significant programs of clinical research and public health education and to provide up to $400,000 per year of charity care (exclusive of bad debts), to be calculated in accordance with the principles set forth in Statement No. 15 of the Principles and Practices Board of the Health Care Financial Management Association, entitled "Valuation and Financial Statement Presentation of Charity Service and Bad Debts by Institutional Health Care Providers," dated February 1993.

In determining that both Friendly Hills and Facey Foundation were entitled to tax-exempt status, the IRS looked to similar factors, including the following:

- Paying the selling physicians no more than the fair market value of assets sold
- Engaging in a number of exempt activities, including providing emergency or urgent care services without regard to patients' ability to pay and providing charity care
- Conducting significant programs of medical research and health education
- Participating in the Medicare and Medicaid programs in a nondiscriminatory fashion
- Appointing governing boards that were broadly representative of their communities, with no more than 20 percent physician representation
- Paying no more than reasonable compensation for professional services to be provided by the physicians, based largely on capitated payments

In light of these two rulings, in order for an entity resulting from a hospital–physician group affiliation to qualify for tax-exempt status, it must observe the following conditions:

- Pay no more than the fair market value of any assets acquired from the physicians
- Pay no more than reasonable compensation for any professional services to be provided by the physicians
- Have a governing board controlled by representatives from the community at large, with limited physician representation
- Participate in the Medicare and Medicaid programs in a nondiscriminatory manner

Although it may not be necessary to demonstrate all of the other elements in the *Friendly Hills* and *Facey Foundation* rulings (teaching and research programs, open medical staff emergency rooms and/or urgent care centers available to the public without regard to ability to pay, provision of charity care, and so forth), the more of these factors that *are* present, the more likely the IRS is to look favorably on an application for tax-exempt status. One strategy may be to include all or as many factors as possible when originally structuring a transaction so as to obtain an exemption but then eliminate one or more in later years. So long as any such changes are reported and the IRS does not object, tax-exempt status would be preserved.

It is not surprising that Friendly Hills and Facey Foundation obtained tax-exempt status because both of these integrated delivery systems exhibited most if not all of the characteristics of a tax-exempt hospital as required by Revenue Ruling 69-545. As more of these entities seek tax-exempt status, the real issue will be how far the IRS will go in granting such status to entities that exhibit some but not all of the characteristics the IRS viewed favorably in these two rulings.

☐ Corporate Practice of Medicine

Most states have statutes that restrict the practice of certain professions, including medicine, to licensed professionals.[10] Many states also have statutes that prohibit any division of fees or charges by a licensed physician with any other licensed physician or any other person.[11] Penalties for violation either of corporate practice of medicine or fee-splitting sanctions include loss of corporate charter; injunction against further operation; and/or disciplinary action against the physician employee, including loss of license to practice.

Over the years most state courts have held that statutes prohibiting the unlicensed practice of medicine and/or fee splitting also prohibit lay corporations from practicing medicine through physician employees, because such corporations are not natural persons and therefore cannot meet the qualifications for obtaining a license to practice medicine. Even though the physician employees in such situations are licensed professionals, courts generally have prohibited the employment of licensed professionals by lay corporations for a number of public policy considerations that relate to maintaining the integrity of the physician–patient relationship.[12] These considerations include avoiding the commercial exploitation of the practice of medicine, maintaining physician control over professional judgments, and ensuring the undivided loyalty of the physician to the patient.

In most states, these older court decisions have been followed by more recent attorney general opinions to the effect that lay corporations cannot employ physicians to practice medicine.[13] For the most part, however, state enforcement authorities (such as attorney generals and state medical boards) have not actively enforced corporate practice of medicine laws. Many state boards have adopted an informal policy that they will not challenge an otherwise legitimate business relationship between a corporation and a physician on corporate practice of medicine grounds, so long as the physician maintains control over his or her professional judgment. Because a number of physician clinics and group practices around the country for many years have operated without challenge as either for-profit or nonprofit corporations that employ physicians to render professional services, there has been a reluctance to enforce the corporate practice of medicine laws vigorously.

Over the years, most states have adopted statutes that permit the formation of professional corporations, so long as their shareholders are exclusively licensed physicians. These statutes permit the practice of medicine by such professional corporations.[14] At the time of this writing, many other states have adopted statutes that permit the formation of limited liability companies and authorize such entities to employ physicians.[15]

Although the risk of prosecution for a corporate practice of medicine or fee-splitting violation is fairly remote in most states, such prosecutions do occur occasionally.[16] An even greater risk is that one party to a transaction may successfully avoid its contractual obligations to the other party by invoking one or both of these doctrines and having the entire arrangement declared illegal and void. See, for example, *Early Detection Center, Inc. v. Wilson*, 248 Kan. 869, 811 P.2d 860 (1991), in which a physician formerly employed by a lay corporation to provide medical services was not required to observe the non-compete clause in his employment contract because the contract was declared void.

In the context of a hospital–group practice affiliation, a number of safeguards can be followed when structuring the transaction to minimize risk of a violation of either the corporate practice of medicine or fee-splitting laws:

- Whenever possible, physicians should be treated as independent contractors rather than employees.
- If physicians are to be employed, they should be employed through a professional corporation.
- A hospital should not participate directly in any professional revenues generated by the physicians. The hospital, however, can be paid by the physicians for leased space or equipment or for management services, so long as the amounts paid are commercially reasonable in light of their value to the physicians.

- Payments based on a percentage of the professional revenues generated by physicians should be avoided.
- Transaction documentation should provide that all matters of professional judgment will be left to the physicians.

One useful technique in hospital–group practice affiliations is the trust/professional corporation model referred to in chapter 3. With this arrangement, the hospital enters into a trust agreement that creates a trust pursuant to which the hospital (or an affiliate) is the beneficiary and a physician or physicians are designated to act as trustee (the physician trustee). The hospital deposits into the trust the capital necessary to fund the affiliation. The trust agreement provides that the physician trustee serves at the pleasure of the hospital and may be removed and/or replaced by the hospital at any time for any reason. The hospital then causes the incorporation of a professional corporation, with the physician trustee as the sole or majority shareholder on behalf of the trust.

Through the physician trustee, the trust purchases shares in the professional corporation and/or makes loan to the corporation in an amount sufficient to capitalize it. The physician trustee, as shareholder of the professional corporation, elects its board of directors, which in turn appoints its officers. Subject to applicable state law, officers and directors may be nonprofessionals from the hospital's board and/or management. The professional corporation then owns and operates the group practice, employs the physicians, and bills and collects all revenues from the operation of the practice. All net revenues, after payment of all operating expenses including physician compensation, can be distributed back to the trust in the form of dividends. In turn the trust can distribute any such net revenues back to the hospital (or its affiliate) as distributions of trust income to the beneficiary. Physician employees can be given the opportunity to become shareholders in the professional corporation.

☐ Antitrust

Less than 20 years ago, health care providers were largely exempt from federal antitrust scrutiny. Today, federal antitrust enforcement agencies have targeted the health care industry as a priority in their investigations and prosecutions.

Although a number of federal and state antitrust statutes must be followed when structuring a hospital–physician group practice affiliation, three federal statutes are most likely to apply: Section 1 of the Sherman Act (15 U.S.C. § 1), which prohibits contracts, combinations, or conspiracies in restraint of trade; Section 2 of the Sherman Act (15 U.S.C. § 2), which prohibits monopolies or attempts to monopolize; and Section 7 of the Clayton Act (15 U.S.C. § 18), which prohibits stock or asset acquisitions, the effect of which is to substantially lessen competition or to tend to create a monopoly.

Penalties for violations of these antitrust statutes are severe. Prosecution for Sherman Act violations may be criminal and civil in nature. Each *criminal* violation is punishable by no more than three years' imprisonment and fines of no more than $350,000 for individuals and $10,000,000 for corporations. The United States Sentencing Guidelines ensure a substantial period of incarceration and a substantial fine for criminal violations of the Sherman Act. Federal enforcement agencies may bring *civil* actions to enjoin violations and to recover damages. Private plaintiffs may also bring such civil actions. A successful lawsuit could result in treble damages and require defendants to pay plaintiffs' attorney fees.

The impact of these federal antitrust laws on a hospital–physician group practice affiliation depends on the facts and circumstances involved in each case. Because of the complex nature of the economic analysis involved in applying these statutes to such affiliations, competent antitrust counsel should review the implications of specific facts of any such affiliation. As a general matter, however, there are two aspects of the typical hospital–group practice affiliation that could have significant antitrust implications: the formation of a combination of physician group practices and the affiliation between that combined practice and the hospital.

Formation of Combined Group Practice

A first step in many hospital–physician group practice affiliations is to combine previously independent physicians and physician groups into one large physician group practice. The primary antitrust issue in this context is whether such combination constitutes an attempt to substantially lessen competition and/or create a monopoly in violation of Section 2 of the Sherman Act and/or Section 7 of the Clayton Act. The merger of physician practices involves the consolidation of competitors in the same line of business (also referred to as a *horizontal merger*). To determine the antitrust implications of such a merger, three elements must be defined: the relevant product market involved, the relevant geographic market for that product, and the impact that the proposed merger will have on market power.

Product Market
In defining the appropriate product line of a combination of physician group practices, not only must physician services be considered in general, but other service areas also must be taken into account. These include specialty services (family practice, obstetrics/gynecology, pediatrics, internal medicine, urology, surgery, and so forth), subspecialty services (cardiovascular surgery, thoracic surgery, orthopedic surgery, and so forth), and ancillary services (diagnostic imaging and laboratory services, for example).

Geographic Market
In defining the relevant geographic market for a particular product line of combined physician practices, the geographic patterns by which medical care is delivered in the area must be examined. This examination also must include population and patient origin statistics.

Market Power
Once the relevant product and geographic markets have been defined, how the proposed merger will bear on market power can be determined. This determination is made in light of the market concentration for particular specialties and/or ancillary services in the relevant geographic market. Federal enforcement agencies have developed what is known as the *Herfindahl–Hirschman Index,* which measures market concentration before and after a proposed combination. The higher the market concentration, the more likely the combination will be challenged.

Absent the formation of a true joint venture among the physicians, many activities undertaken between them (such as fixing prices and/or dividing markets) may be deemed illegal *per se* under the antitrust laws, meaning that such activities are deemed to have no *pro*competition aspects and that merely engaging in them is illegal. By comparison, activities that are not considered illegal per se are viewed under a rule-of-reason analysis, that is, whether the procompetition aspects of the activities outweigh their *anti*competition effects.

Affiliation between Physician Group Practice and Hospital

When a hospital–physician group practice affiliation is proposed, the issue presented is whether this combination will result in a substantial lessening of competition, restraint of trade, or an attempt to monopolize. To the extent that the hospital and physicians previously competed with one another (for example, in the providing of certain ancillary services such as diagnostic imaging), the same type of market analysis must be undertaken as described with respect to combining physician practices. The other crucial issue is whether such combination will constitute a genuine joint venture.

The leading case in this area is *Arizona v. Maricopa County Medical Society*, 457 U.S. 332 (1982). Maricopa Foundation for Medical Care was organized as a nonprofit corporation to promote fee-for-service medical care and to provide a competitive alternative to existing health insurance plans. The foundation performed three primary activities: it established a maximum fee schedule for participating physicians to accept as payment in full for patients insured under plans approved by the foundation; reviewed the medical necessity and appropriateness of treatment provided by its members; and paid physicians out of insurance company accounts for covered services. The U.S. Supreme Court ruled the fee schedule per se illegal price fixing. The Court refused to consider whether the fee schedule had any positive effects on the relevant market and rejected the argument that the foundation was analogous to a partnership or joint venture because it did not involve pooling of capital and shared risk of loss.

Depending on the nature of the activity to be undertaken in a hospital–physician group affiliation, it may be necessary to qualify such affiliation as a true economic joint venture so as to avoid antitrust issues. Doing so requires hospital and physicians to pool capital and share risk for substantial loss. These requirements could be satisfied by requiring a substantial financial contribution from the physicians and/or proof of true risk sharing, for example, by significant withholds of payment as part of a capitated payment system.

New Antitrust Safety Zones

Recognizing the dilemma created for hospitals and physicians seeking to affiliate in an atmosphere of escalating legal risks, the Department of Justice and the Federal Trade Commission jointly announced (in a policy statement issued September 15, 1993) six "antitrust safety zones" for health care providers. According to the agencies, these zones are intended "to resolve, as completely as possible, the problem of antitrust uncertainties that some have said may deter mergers or joint ventures that would lower health care costs." The agencies further declare that "as a matter of prosecutorial discretion," they will not make an antitrust challenge in defined circumstances in the following areas: hospital mergers, hospital joint ventures involving high technology or other expensive equipment, physicians' provision of information to purchasers of health care services, hospital participation in exchanges of price and cost information, joint purchasing arrangements among health care providers, and physician network joint ventures. Two of these safety zones, physicians' provision of information to purchasers of health care services and physician network joint ventures, could apply to at least certain aspects of a hospital–group practice affiliation.

Physicians' Provision of Information to Purchasers of Health Care Services
This safety zone applies to physicians who collectively (for example, through a medical society) give underlying medical data relating to the mode, quality, or efficiency of treatment. For example, physicians may give outcome data from a certain procedure and also develop "suggested" practice parameters to assist in clinical decision making. Physicians may not, however, attempt to coerce purchasers by threatening to boycott plans that do not follow their joint recommendation. The safety zone also does not apply to collective action by physicians to assemble and provide fee-related information to purchasers or to exchange such information among competing physicians.

Physician Network Joint Ventures
This safety zone is intended to apply to networks such as IPAs and PPOs. Federal enforcement agencies will not challenge a network of participating physicians who (1) constitute 20 percent or less of the physicians in each specialty with active hospital staff privileges

in the relevant geographic market and (2) share substantial financial risk. *Substantial financial risk* in the agencies' view requires either an agreement to provide service at a capitated rate or financial incentives such as withholds to encourage and reward cost-containment achievements.

Health care providers do not necessarily violate the antitrust laws, and will not necessarily be challenged, if they engage in conduct that falls outside these safety zones. Unfortunately, the safety zones are narrow and offer little protection for many aspects of the typical hospital–physician group practice affiliation. They do, however, indicate recognition on the part of federal enforcers of the dilemma facing health care providers that try to structure such arrangements. Such recognition may represent a first step toward a more realistic approach to enforcement activity.

☐ Employee Benefit Plans

Because most hospitals and physicians participate in employee benefit plans of one type or another, an important issue during affiliation negotiations is what impact affiliation may have on the plans. Employers often seek to have their plans "qualified" under Section 401(a) of the Code in order to enjoy certain tax benefits and other advantages associated with qualified plans. Benefits include a current deduction for amounts the employer contributed to the plan, the certainty that benefits are funded through a trust that earns tax-free income, and the assurance that plan participants do not recognize income on account of plan contributions or earnings until they actually receive plan benefits.

A qualified retirement plan that loses its qualified status imposes severe consequences, including participants becoming subject to current federal income tax on plan contributions made subsequent to this qualification and the loss of tax-exempt status for the trust through which plan benefits are funded.

Under the right circumstances, a nonqualified plan can be an effective means of providing deferred compensation, whether by salary deferrals or otherwise. Nonqualified plans are generally maintained for the benefit of highly compensated employees. The reason for this has to do with certain funding requirements under the code and the 1974 Employee Retirement Income Security Act (ERISA), as amended, which provide that a plan must be funded unless it is maintained solely for a selected group of managers or highly compensated employees. However, unless the benefits of a nonqualified plan are subject to a "substantial risk of forfeiture" (which generally means that receipt of benefits is conditioned on the future performance of substantial services), plan contributions can result in current income to plan participants under the constructive receipt rule. This rule attributes income to a person under certain circumstances, even though the person is not in actual receipt of the income, resulting in potential income tax liability but no cash.

For these reasons, most employers operate nonqualified plans on an "unfunded" basis. Alternatively, some nonqualified plans are set up through what the IRS refers to as *rabbi trusts,* that is, trust assets are available to the employers' creditors and therefore are not deemed to have been received by the employee until actually distributed.

A plan must satisfy three basic tests to be qualified under the Code: the nondiscrimination test of Section 401(a)(4), the participation test of Section 401(a)(26), and the coverage test of Section 410(b). Depending on the nature of the affiliation, these tests may be applied on a consolidated basis to the plans of the hospital and physician group practice participating in an affiliation under the controlled group and separate line of business rules.

Nondiscrimination Test

The *nondiscrimination test* requires that a plan not discriminate in favor of highly compensated employees with respect to plan contributions, benefits, rights, or features. Regulations under Section 401(a)(4) of the Code provide certain safe harbors that a plan can satisfy with respect to benefits or contributions. The safe harbors establish a permitted range of disparity as to those benefits accrued or contributions made in favor of highly compensated employees versus benefits or contributions that favor non–highly compensated employees.

Participation Test

The *participation test* requires that a plan benefit the lesser of 50 employees or 40 percent of all employees of an employer. As discussed more fully below, because the participation test is applied to plans on a consolidated basis in the case of employers in a controlled group of corporations, the participation requirement often makes it difficult for a small employer and a controlled group of larger employers to offer a separate qualified plan. However, as of this writing legislation is pending in Congress that would modify Section 401(a)(26) of the Code to make it applicable only to certain defined benefit plans maintained by an employer.

Coverage Test

The *coverage test* is relatively simple. It is satisfied if the percentage of non–highly compensated employees who benefit under a plan is at least 70 percent of the percentage of highly compensated employees who benefit.

Controlled Group Rules

Controlled group rules provide that whenever a group of corporations are related by common ownership or control, the qualified plans of such entities must be tested on a consolidated basis to determine whether plans can maintain their qualified status. When a qualified plan maintained by a small employer in a controlled group with one or more large employers is tested on a consolidated basis, it can be difficult for the plan of the small employer to satisfy the nondiscrimination, participation, and coverage standards described above.

When plans within a controlled group are tested on a consolidated basis, each individual employer within the group is treated as employing all of the employees of all employers within the group. The result is that, for test purposes, an individual employer ends up with a larger "workforce," making it more difficult for that employer's plan to satisfy the tests for qualified status.

Separate Line of Business Rules

Separate line of business rules provide an exception to the consolidated testing of plans of employers of a controlled group. Under these rules, if an employer operates a line of business organized and operated separately from its other activities, with separate financial accountability, a separate employee workforce, separate management, and at least 50 employees, and if the line of business passes "administrative scrutiny," then a plan maintained by this separate line of business can be tested separately from any other plans maintained by other members of the controlled group for purposes of determining whether the plan maintained by the separate line of business is a qualified plan. The phrase *passing administrative scrutiny* means that the separate line of business satisfies either a statutory safe harbor for determining whether a line of business is a qualified separate line of business or certain guidelines prescribed in IRS regulations.

Generally speaking, an entity will constitute a separate line of business if it operates as a separate organizational unit, maintains its own financial books and records providing for separate revenue and expense information, has a separate workforce, has its own management team, and has its own tangible assets. To qualify as a separate line of business, the entity must also have at least 50 employees and pass administrative scrutiny. If these conditions are satisfied, upon giving of notice to the IRS, the entity may qualify as a separate line of business.

The separate line of business rules will not avoid the consolidated testing requirements if entities that are members of the controlled group are also part of an "affiliated service group." This would be the case if it were determined that two or more entities in the controlled group are regularly associated with one another in the performance of services for third parties, or if one entity derives a significant portion (that is, 10 percent or more) of its revenues from performing services for one of the other members of the controlled group.

In the context of a hospital–physician group practice affiliation, it is probable that prior to the affiliation the practice has maintained a qualified plan that is more generous than the qualified plan maintained by the hospital and its related entities. In this situation a careful analysis must be performed of the terms of the respective plans and of the facts and circumstances of the affiliation to determine whether qualified status can be maintained for the different plans in light of the tests described above. If the affiliation results in the hospital and the physicians being in a controlled group or affiliated service group, it may not be possible to maintain the qualified status of the physicians' plan. In that event, adopting a nonqualified plan is an alternative. Otherwise, the parties will have to weigh the cost of losing qualified plan status in their cost–benefit analysis of determining whether to proceed with the proposed affiliation.

☐ Conclusion

Although it is clear that the formation of integrated delivery systems between hospitals and physicians will become a crucial option in light of changes in the health care marketplace, it is equally clear that such affiliations raise serious legal issues. This chapter identified the most important of these issues and various ways to address them, but it will be difficult if not impossible to completely eliminate all risk associated with these legal issues in the context of a specific hospital–physician group affiliation. All parties should consider the techniques described in this chapter so as to minimize risks, but they should also recognize that proceeding with the transactions described here involve a certain amount of inherent risk. Benefits of the proposed transaction must be weighed against the risks so that an informed business decision can be made as to whether to proceed. Where an affiliation is implemented between a hospital and a physician group, future legal developments affecting the issues discussed here should be monitored carefully. Then all concerned should adapt their relationships as appropriate.

References

1. 42 U.S.C. § 1320a-7b.

2. See, for example, California Business & Professional Code § 650, and Ohio Revised Code § 3999.22.

3. See *United States v. Greber*, 760 F.2d 68, Cert. denied, 474 U.S. 988 (1985); *United States v. Kats*, 871 F.2d 105 (1989); and *United States v. Bay State Ambulance and Hospital Rental Service, Inc.*, 874 F.2d 20 (1989).

4. See 42 U.S.C. § 1320a-7b(b)(3).

5. 42 U.S.C. § 1395nn.

6. *Internal Revenue Manual*, 7751, Exempt Organizations Handbook, § 381.1.

7. See General Counsel Memorandum 39498.

8. For examples of this scrutiny, see *Lowry Hospital Association v. Commissioner,* 66 TC 850 (1976) and *Harding Hospital v. United States,* 505 F.2d 1068 (6th Cir. 1974).

9. See General Counsel Memorandum 39862.

10. See, for example, Ohio R. C. § 4731.41 and 63 Pa. Cons. Stat. § 421.3.

11. See, for example, Ohio R. C. § 4731.22(B)(17).

12. See, for example, *Parker v. Board of Dental Examiners,* 216 Cal. 185, 14 F.2d 67 (1932).

13. See, for example, Ohio Op. Atty. Gen. No. 1751 (1952) and 30 Pa. Dist. R. 778.

14. See, for example, Ohio R. C. § 1785.01 *et. seq.* and 15 Pa. Cons. Stat. § 2901 *et seq.*

15. See, for example, Ohio R. C. § 1705.01 *et. seq.*

16. See, for example, *California Association of Disposing Opticians v. Pearle Vision Center,* 145 Cal. App.3d 419, 191 Cal. Rptr. 762 (1983).

Part Two

Case Studies

Introduction to Part Two

Criteria for the selection of case studies were developed with three objectives in mind. The first was to present the variety of circumstances that can lead to a hospital–group practice affiliation; the second was to provide a closer look at the organizational structures presented in chapter 3; and the third was to offer examples of how various business, legal, and organizational issues affect the affiliation effort. Some of the criteria used to select organizations for case studies include the following:

- *Experience:* This category shows what impact the affiliation has on the hospital and physician group. Also, the affiliated entities chosen for these case studies have completed at least one year's operating experience under their structure.
- *Motivations for affiliation:* A full range of hospital and physician needs and motivations are reflected throughout the case studies.
- *Physician group composition and size:* Examples include hospitals that joined with existing physician groups as well as those that created new group practices through integration of existing practices or recruitment of new physicians. Primary care physician groups as well as multispecialty groups are included. Group size ranges from 3 to more than 50 physicians.
- *New or freestanding group practices:* Group practices and hospitals with a long history of affiliation are not included. Although entities such as the Cleveland Clinic or the Mayo Clinic, for example, represent strong models of integrated systems, the hospital–physician culture that has evolved over time in these organizations is not easily duplicated in affiliations of previously independent or newly created group practices and community hospitals.
- *Affiliation structure:* Criteria for the cases included an affiliation that involved, at minimum, hospital ownership of practice assets and responsibility for practice management services. Less integrated organizational structures, such as hospital practice enhancement services or PHOs, do not reflect the variety of issues raised in developing a more integrated physician group–hospital affiliation.
- *Health care environment:* The case studies represent a variety of health care environments. These include, but are not limited to, urban (versus rural) settings; single-hospital communities (versus multihospital competitive environments); varying

levels of managed care penetration in the market; and dominance of solo (versus group) medical practices in the market.

More than 50 hospital–group practice affiliations were reviewed while researching material for this book. Aside from the criteria previously listed, organizations were selected based on their willingness and ability to devote the time and energy needed to develop a comprehensive case study. Another important consideration was the lesson(s) to be learned from each experience.

The cases represent a unique set of circumstances from which affiliation structures emerged through a planning and negotiation process designed to accommodate those circumstances. Both research and the evidence presented reinforce the fact that no generic structure can be "pulled from the shelf" when integration is indicated. The process of understanding hospital and physician motivations, the changing health care environment in which they exist, the business and legal issues that affect the prospective affiliation, and the mutual goals to be achieved is the route to intelligent negotiations that lead to a successful affiliation.

The histories shared here are the result of trial-and-error collaborative strategies. The authors of each case study indicated the intent to further modify their organizations' structures and operations in a continued effort to improve on the integration.

The following table presents the key elements introduced with each case study. These elements provide a backdrop summary of what is to follow in each narrative.

Case Study Elements

Affiliated Practice(s) Characteristics	Midwest Medical Center	Mercy Healthcare Sacramento, CA	Good Samaritan Foundation San Jose, CA	Millard Fillmore Health Center Buffalo, NY	Mercy Hospital Pittsburgh, PA	St. Luke's Hospital Saginaw, MI	Monroe Clinic Monroe, WI
Single specialty	X			X	X	X	
Multispecialty		X	X				X
Number of Doctors							
1–5						X	
6–10		X			X		
10–20	X			X			
20 +		X	X				X
Management Services							
Centralized	X	X	X	X	X		X
Decentralized						X	
Combination							
Group Practice							
Existing prior to affiliation		X	X				X
New				X	X	X	
Combination	X						
Age							
0–2 years		X	X				X
3–5 years	X					X	
5 years +				X	X		
Structure							
MSO/hospital-owned practice assets	X						
Foundation model/contract with physician group		X	X				
Trust/professional corporation	X						
Hospital-owned practice—contracted physician services				X			
Hospital-owned practice—direct physician employment					X	X	X
Physician Compensation							
Salary				X	X		
Production	X						X
Salary and incentive						X	
Bottom line		X	X				
Capitated Reimbursement Percent							
0–20%	X			X	X		X
21–50%						X	
51% +		X	X				

Chapter 6
Midwest Medical Center

☐ Executive Summary: Key Elements of the Affiliation

- *Organizational structure:* A hospital MSO provides assets and complete management services to physician practices, including a freestanding internal medicine group practice formed to purchase the practices of retiring physicians and employ new recruits.

- *Hospital goals:* Midwest Medical Center (MMC) had the short-term need to protect the practices of retiring primary care physicians from sale and transition to physicians loyal to competitor hospitals. The hospital also recognized the long-term strategic need to develop a primary care base for its hospital, both to maintain patient volume and to contract with managed care insurers.

- *Physician needs and goals:* Retiring primary care physicians sought to sell and facilitate transition of their practices. Surgeons and subspecialists on the medical staff endorsed development and enhancement of the primary care referral sources.

- *Personal relationships:* The key relationship in the development of this group was between the hospital and a respected internist who became sole owner of the group practice.

- *Health care reform and managed care:* Neither MMC's market nor its medical staff had experienced significant impact from health care reform or the introduction of insurance products that reimburse physicians on a capitated basis.

- *Market and competitor activity:* Competitor hospitals were aggressively seeking to acquire practices of physicians loyal to MMC. The community did not have an identified need for additional primary care physicians, which affected MMC's ability to recruit additional physicians.

- *Capital needs and resources:* Midwest Medical Center had established an MSO that also provided operating support to medical practices. Capital was required to acquire the hard assets of existing practices. Loans were provided to the new group practice physician owner to acquire the practices and employ physicians. The start-up budget was based on a business plan developed with the help of outside consultants.

The name of the hospital depicted in this case has been changed to a fictitious one.

113

- *Physician recruitment and retention:* The hospital–group practice affiliation proved to be a successful vehicle for recruitment of existing physicians and several physicians new to the area to take over the practices of retiring physicians.
- *Legal and contractual issues:* Midwest Medical Center needed to address the legal issues of the corporate practice of medicine laws. Contracts with the physicians, including the basis of incentive compensation, have been modified to conform to the goals and needs of the group.

☐ Introduction

In the mid-1980s, Midwest Medical Center (MMC) became aware of a number of pending retirements in its internal medicine department. In responding to the need for transition and revitalization of existing practices, as well as protection against losing practices to competitor institutions, MMC created a practice management company and an affiliated group practice to purchase, integrate, and expand practices of internists on its medical staff who were near retirement. The group experienced rapid growth (14 physicians) in two years. The hospital's success in developing a group practice through offering a positive alternative to retiring physicians was well beyond its expectations.

Although the primary objective was achieved, numerous operational and financial problems arose as a result of such rapid growth. Despite difficult and time-consuming corrective actions, MMC developed a solid base of practice management expertise as well as a strongly affiliated primary care group practice to serve as the cornerstone in its strategy to become a fully integrated health care organization.

☐ Background

Health care is a major sphere of economic influence in MMC's city, an urban area with more than 47 hospitals providing care to a population of 2,700,000. Health care providers in the area include several nationally recognized centers of excellence and major training facilities, but few group practices.

Throughout the 1980s managed care had relatively little impact in the metropolitan area. There were no significant capitated products, and physicians were reimbursed based primarily on a discounted fee-for-service schedule. However, increased market penetration by several national managed care organizations has caused the number of patients covered under capitation to rise significantly. This trend is anticipated to continue.

In addition, an adequate number of physicians were available to the community in the mid-1980s. New physicians required significant time and start-up capital to develop a patient base that could support new practices, and although many physicians preferred the autonomy of solo practice, the time it took to become self-sustaining was longer than anticipated. Because of this, new physicians sought group practice positions.

The hospital environment has also been very competitive. Since the early 1980s, many hospitals interested in expanding their inpatient business have offered lucrative and aggressive support packages to new physicians who purchase or join an established practice. Thus, MMC has been faced with the loss of admissions and referrals to competitor hospitals from formerly loyal practices.

The Hospital's Response to Managed Care

Midwest Medical Center is a 450-bed hospital located in a low-income urban setting in close proximity to a large university hospital. Despite this location, MMC draws most of its patients from its city's affluent eastern suburbs, where its medical staff practices are located. In 1986, hospital administrators launched a strategic planning process, with input and support from its board and medical staff. The goal was to establish long-term strategies to address the growth of managed care in the area and the anticipated shift of services to an ambulatory setting. This plan identified the services necessary to meet the community's future health care needs. In the past, MMC had been successful in building its clinical services around the recruitment of preeminent specialists. The strategic plan, however, identified the need for a strong primary care base.

Other strategic initiatives included developing satellite ancillary services throughout the community, because MMC discovered that its outpatient-to-inpatient service ratio did not correlate with that of other similar institutions. Satellite offices for the laboratory, X-ray, and other ancillary departments were established in medical office buildings. In December 1993 a 200,000-square-foot satellite campus that incorporated physician offices, hospital ancillary service satellites, and an ambulatory surgery center was opened in the eastern suburbs.

The hospital has grown through the acquisition of a freestanding mental health and substance abuse facility and the development of other community outpatient facilities. For example, a full-service occupational and environmental program was established in response to identified needs of employers throughout the community. Hoping to gain a competitive edge as managed care penetration expanded, MMC sought to establish positive relationships with businesses based on the quality of medical services it provided.

Medical Staff

In the mid-1980s, the majority of physicians on Midwest's medical staff practiced solo or in small groups of two or three physicians. The medical staff was dominated by specialists. Demands from MMC's nonspecialist staff for facilities and equipment was the dominant issue between hospital administrators and medical staff. Among physicians, relationships revolved mostly around referral patterns. With the need to shift focus toward primary care in order to develop a health care delivery system that would attract insurers and industries in the future, strong primary care relationships were considered essential.

Physicians, aware of competing hospital support for medical practices, wanted MMC to provide similar support to its medical staff. These requests included: financial assistance in practice expansion and new physician recruitment; management assistance in managed care contract negotiations and practice operation; and retirement assistance that included identification of physicians who desired to purchase the practices of retiring physicians, as well as financial support to the new physicians during practice transition.

In 1987, the average age of physicians in the internal medicine department was 53, with 32 percent of the department over age 60. These senior physicians accounted for 34 percent of MMC's internal medicine admissions. Despite the existence of a family medicine department, well over 70 percent of MMC's primary care admissions were made by internists.

Physicians nearing retirement were experiencing difficulty in identifying younger successors to the practices they had built over the past 30 years. Many senior physicians had planned on their practice sale proceeds being a major component of their retirement savings. Competitor hospitals were approaching these physicians with aggressive proposals to sell the practices to younger physicians supported by those hospitals. Several internal medicine physicians, although traditionally loyal to MMC, found these offers so attractive they considered them their only viable alternative.

Two circumstances contributed to MMC's difficulty in helping to recruit new physicians who could match the needs of senior physicians. First, based on a conservative interpretation of the laws and regulations governing physician–hospital relationships, MMC was limited in the options it had to offer. Second, MMC found the younger physicians' interests to be incompatible with the retiring physicians' plans. For example, graduating residents wanted to act quickly—purchase the practice, transfer patients and their records, and retire the selling physician. On the contrary, senior physicians wanted to be more methodical. Not only were these senior physicians adjusting to the concept of retirement, but also they wanted their patients transferred to a quality-conscious and

115

concerned physician. In essence, senior physicians desired a transition period of several years. Furthermore, they were in a position to compare MMC proposals to offers for the purchase of their practices from physicians sponsored by MMC competitors.

Hospital Practice Management Services

Midwest Healthcare Management, Inc. (MHM), a for-profit subsidiary of MMC, was established in 1983. Initially MHM had owned and operated a network of urgent care centers. In July 1988, Midwest Practice Management Company (MPMC) was created as a division of MHM to provide support to physician practices.

The mission of this division was to provide management and financial services for practices established as part of the MMC primary care physician recruitment and retention objectives. Specifically, the division provided office space leasing, practice personnel leasing, billing services, marketing support, management services, financial services, and consulting to medical practices. The company was paid a fair and reasonable fee, either in the form of a flat monthly fee or a percentage of practice revenues. Quickly MPMC entered into several contracts with physician practices.

☐ The Planning Initiative

Upon further study of the pending retirements from the internal medicine department, MMC administrators determined that a creative effort was needed. Because young physicians were hesitant to purchase solo practices and instead were seeking to join group practices, and because 90 percent of the senior physicians operated solo practices, the hospital concluded that the development of a group practice would provide the best vehicle for protecting its primary care base, attracting new primary care physicians, and responding to the needs of the retiring physicians.

The hospital and medical staff (including specialists) were motivated by four mutual objectives:

1. To develop a loyal, high-quality primary care group practice to address the current and future health care environment
2. To preempt the hospital's eroding primary care base
3. To improve the hospital's market position, as well as that of its specialty staff, through the transition and revitalization of primary care practices
4. To establish an opportunity for group practice for young primary care physicians

Once this strategic plan was accepted by the parties, the hospital moved forward with its planning initiative. At about this time, a prominent internist on MMC's medical staff who operated a successful two-physician practice expressed interest in developing a group practice. The hospital immediately approached this physician (who subsequently became the physician leader) to discuss development of a primary care group practice. After evaluating alternatives, including the creation of a professional corporation held in physician-controlled trust for the hospital, it was agreed that the practice would be owned by the physician and that MPMC (the hospital's management company) would oversee its operations. Consultants were brought in to work with the planning team, which consisted of the physician leader and MMC's senior vice-president for corporate development, in setting up a structure and business plan for the group practice.

Medical Staff Reaction

In presenting the plan for a group practice to its medical staff in 1988, the planning team stressed the key objectives—especially the importance of protecting and expanding the primary care base and the hospital support available to its physicians. This support included management services, recruitment assistance, and education on addressing practice-related managed care contracting issues.

Specialty and surgical staff endorsed the initiative, but when the internal medicine department balked, its senior physicians—who comprised the department's informal leadership—carried the plan through. Many of the younger physicians, however, concerned over lack of opportunity, were reassured when the team reiterated the management support available to them and the group practice opportunity.

Issues, Success Strategies, and Plan Approval

The formalized plan for developing a primary care group practice was presented to the boards of the hospital and MHM. The planning team reviewed a list of critical issues and development strategies with the boards. This list included the following:

- Creating a compelling proposal package for senior primary care physicians to join the group
- Utilizing a physician leader, respected for his clinical acumen and medical practice experience, in developing the group practice
- Developing a fair market value approach for the purchase of existing practices
- Providing equity opportunity in the practice for young physician recruits
- Providing physician financial incentives related to practice revenues
- Retaining senior physicians in their practices during transition to the new group practice location and patient transfer

The critical issues and strategies for successful implementation of a primary care group practice at MMC were accepted by the boards. Next, detailed planning and negotiation was undertaken by the hospital's senior vice-president of corporate development, MHM managers, and the group physician leader.

Consultants provided estimates (based on medical staff interviews) on the number of physicians who would join the group through practice acquisitions and recruitment. Projected growth assumption, which took into account retiring and newly recruited physicians, was eight physicians during the first three years (1990–1993), with new recruits offsetting the retired physicians.

The consultant assisted in the development of a business plan that included projected patient volumes, revenues, and expenses for the group practice. Strategies and valuation approaches for negotiation of practice purchases and an implementation schedule, including assignment of responsibilities and time frames, were established by the planning team.

Options for Organizational Structure

The state where MMC is located has a corporate practice of medicine law restricting the ownership of medical practices by nonphysicians. The restriction includes hospitals, so two alternatives were investigated to address this legal issue surrounding the planned purchase of retiring physicians' practices.

One option was to develop a professional corporation whose stock would be owned by the hospital but held in trust by a physician selected by the hospital for his or her loyalty to MMC. The physician would not need to participate actively in the practice; the trust arrangement would provide for the medical practice to be in the hands of a licensed physician and would comply with state regulations. The professional corporation would buy the intangible assets of the practices and employ the physicians.

The second option was to establish a professional corporation owned by the selected physician leader of the group and support his or her investment in purchasing the intangible assets of the practices and start-up costs for the group through interest-bearing loans from the hospital. Again, loyalty to the hospital would be a key factor in selecting the physician owner, who would be involved in the practice.

With either alternative, MHM would purchase the practices' hard assets, employ the nonphysician staff, and provide all management support, while the physician-controlled professional corporation would purchase the practices' goodwill and employ the physicians. Not only did both options address the corporate practice of medicine laws, they were more consistent with Medicare fraud and abuse proscriptions and IRS private inurement regulations. Neither the tax-exempt hospital nor its subsidiary would purchase the "goodwill value" of a retiring physician's practice.

Because the lead physician wished to retain ownership of the practice, the second structure was selected for the new group practice. The trust approach (illustrated in figure 6-1) was used by MMC in subsequent practice purchases not affiliated with the group.

☐ Negotiations

Upon entering negotiations, the hospital knew that the physician owner had a very productive practice, and therefore the hospital wanted to ensure that his efforts in purchasing practices, recruiting new physicians, and developing a group practice would be rewarded in a way that offset the loss in productivity and income his practice would experience. In addition, because group practice management was a new element of MPMC's medical practices services, it was agreed that the physician would provide leadership for the practice operations.

Negotiations led to agreement that, in addition to continued income from his practice activities, the physician owner would be paid a base salary for administrative activities and a bonus based on each practice purchase successfully negotiated and integrated

Figure 6-1. MMC's Structure for Practice Acquisition

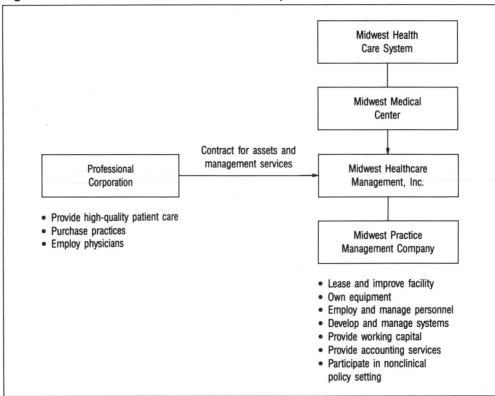

into the group. The expense for this base salary and bonus package would be considered operating expenses for the practice and paid by MPMC.

Further negotiation established the fee for MPMC services to the practice at 50 percent of net practice revenues. The professional corporation would pay 80 percent of the net revenue (40 percent of total revenue) to the physician employees of the group based on their individual practice productivity. Remaining revenue (10 percent of total revenue) would be used to conduct the corporation's business and repay loans received for purchase of intangible assets and employment of physicians.

The physician owner signed a contract, and the new professional corporation was formed with the contribution of his existing practice assets. The physician owner and his associates retained their practice accounts receivables. Legal documents setting forth the formation of the professional corporation were prepared and approved for the new group, which was to be named Internal Medicine Group.

☐ Implementation

Once the professional corporation was formed and implementation details worked out, the new group practice began to take shape. As physician growth progressed, issues surrounding practice operations began to surface. Among these considerations were practice location, valuation and acquisition terms, physician contracts, organizational structure, compensation, number of physicians and patient volume, and the transition from an independent operations mentality to a group focus.

Practice Location

The new practice was located in an affluent suburb, an area optimally suited to the practices targeted for purchase and to the hospital's market area. The specific site was a medical office building where a number of MMC physicians and services already were located. The cost of the space was high but was offset by the accessibility and quality of the site.

Practice Valuations and Acquisition Terms

The value of intangible assets of the practices purchased was determined using formulas developed by MMC. The values, which were averaged and compared to industry standards to determine a fair market value for each practice, were accepted by the physician owner of Internal Medicine Group. The elements of each practice valuation included the following:

- Practice revenues and practice profits applied to net-present-value calculations
- Comparison to national norms for similar practices (revenues, volumes, expenses, and so forth)
- Number of active charts
- Payer mix
- Patient demographics
- Projected patient retention in the practice

Hard assets were assigned a fair market value through application of industry standards, based on their replacement values and useful lives. Again, this value was established by MMC and accepted by the physician owner.

Existing accounts receivable were retained by the physician whose practice was purchased. In several of the initial purchases, MHM agreed to collect these receivables on behalf of the physician for a nominal fee. This proved to be a source of conflict between physicians and the management company: Physicians were dissatisfied with collection efforts, which caused some loss of credibility for MHM. In fact, collections were reasonable based on their age and the information available from the practice but did not meet physician expectations. This service was discontinued in the first year.

Physician Contracts

Retiring physicians were not restricted as to the length of time they would remain in practice. Some were hired "at will," while others, whose retirement was imminent, signed five-year employment contracts. Physicians maintained independence in determining their practice patterns relative to scheduling and staffing. Despite an anticipated slowdown in their practice activities, they were guaranteed space equivalent to the number of examination rooms and offices they had throughout their private practice years. Nonphysician staff members of these practices were offered employment at MPMC at their current salary rates. Employee benefits typically were better at MPMC than they had been at the respective practices.

Group Practice Organization

Midwest Medical Center developed no group practice management expertise. Traditionally, medical practice management support had been provided to solo practitioners under the physician's control. Initially MPMC was structured to provide specific physician services and consultation as needed, not comprehensive group practice management. The physician owner's success in a two-physician group practice was assumed to be applicable in a larger group setting. With MPMC's service support, the owner was believed capable of implementing the management systems, policies, and procedures required to transform independent practices into a single-site group practice. As the group evolved, however, these assumptions proved to be unrealistic.

Because of the initial emphasis on purchasing the practices of retiring physicians, the physician owner selected a manager who had previously worked for the hospital in developing laboratory services to meet physician practice needs. The senior vice-president for corporate development expressed concern over the manager's lack of practice experience but deferred to the physician owner. The manager's major strength lay in dealing with physicians and developing positive relationships with personnel, management skills the physician owner felt to be essential. Again, because the manager had no group practice experience, the physician owner was expected to guide practice operations and service direction for the management company.

Physician Compensation

As described earlier, Internal Medicine Group paid its employed physicians who previously had owned the practices purchased by the group a guaranteed 40 percent of total collections generated from their ongoing practice activities. This was determined to be well within the percentage of collections generally earned by internal medicine physicians in the market area. It was believed that a guaranteed percentage of revenues would be incentive enough for the physicians to maintain their practice levels. The retiring physicians were expected to assist in the transition of their patients to the younger physicians, thus maintaining for the group the revenue stream from their practices. It soon became apparent that the physician compensation formula conflicted with this practice transition goal.

Newly hired physicians with no practices were provided a two-year income guarantee by MMC, consistent with its recruitment support program and policies. This guarantee ran counter to practice revenues, and at the end of two years the new hires received compensation under the group's formula of 40 percent of total practice collections.

Number of Group Physicians

Internal Medicine Group initially stabilized at 14 of the 16 physicians assimilated into the group during the first two years. Figure 6-2 charts the actual practice growth over a four-year period. The first 16 physicians to join the group included the physician owner and his associate, both in their mid-40s; 10 physicians over age 60 whose practices were purchased; 3 younger physicians newly recruited to the area; and 1 physician in his mid-40s, who was the associate of a retiring physician.

The group's rapid growth necessitated an increase in office space from approximately 5,600 square feet to 11,200 square feet. As physicians joined, nonphysician staffing increased from 11 to more than 30. The number of active charts increased from the 3,000 originally held by the physician owner and his associate to an excess of 20,000 charts.

Most management attention was devoted to the negotiation, closing, and integration of the practices of retiring physicians. As a result, operating issues sometimes were addressed inadequately. For example, systems fragmentation (physicians continued to practice as if they were minipractices within a large group setting); billing and accounts receivable management systems overload; and lack of teamwork or group practice mentality (detailed in a following section) became problematic.

Patient Volume

Patient volume and revenues failed to keep pace with the number of group physicians. The retiring physicians, after cashing out of their practices, were content to practice at a reduced pace in the new group setting—despite being compensated at a percentage of their practice revenue. Their practice volume decreased, with little transition activity to new physicians. Senior physicians were comfortable and did not want to retire, and the growth of the new physicians' practices was slow. Furthermore, marketing activities for Internal Medicine Group had been limited, because it was presumed that patient volume would expand with the integration of existing practices. In fact, the group experienced patient erosion as physicians moved their practices to the new location. The

Figure 6-2. Planned versus Actual Group Practice Growth (1989–1993)

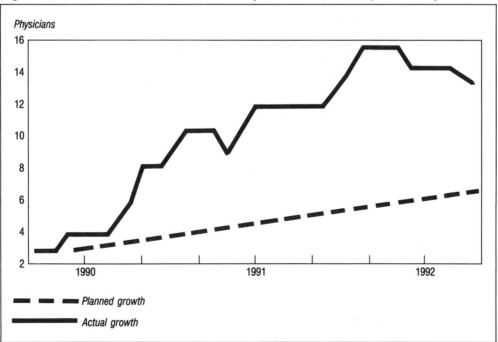

outcome of this combination of events was that original estimates of practice activities relative to active patient charts acquired in practice purchases proved to be overoptimistic.

The Transition from Independent Operation to Group Focus

As mentioned above, the organization failed to function as a group practice. Despite efforts to integrate operations and staff into a coordinated team effort, each practice tended to operate independently. The impact of the physical move, the opening of additional space at Internal Medicine Group, and the orientation of personnel to basic systems in the new practice suffered as a result of inadequate time frames for implementing effective group practice management systems or policies. Furthermore, employees of the purchased practices were concerned about job security under the management company. This lack of trust caused them to resist efforts to change their work habits to accommodate a group environment.

The physician owner continued to operate autonomously, as had been his style with his two-physician practice. Consequently, other physicians were left out of decisions that affected the group. This further exacerbated the propensity among individual physicians to act in their own interests rather than those of the group.

Internal Medicine Group could not meet timetables to correct problems that continued to escalate relative to operational expenses and poor billing and collections. Despite the initial success in identifying and acquiring physician practices and creating a larger-than-expected group in a surprisingly short period of time, the physicians continued to function independently, and many of the projected benefits of a group practice were not achieved.

☐ Outcomes

In late 1992, MHM's board expressed its growing concern over practice operations, specifically with respect to poor collection activities, increasing accounts receivable, and overhead in excess of 80 percent of practice revenues. The computer system, a locally developed software package, had been changed to a more widely known package, but the conversion process was slow and compounded the collection problem. Staff resistance to clinic policies that replaced policies in their old practices became more and more apparent.

The physician owner continued to put most of his energies into practice expansion, for it had become apparent that his interests and strength lay in bringing physicians into the group. He believed that a practice limited to general internists would continue to have difficulty generating revenues to support the expenses of a large group practice effectively; thus, he sought to incorporate medical subspecialists into the group. This created concern among the medical staff that Internal Medicine Group might become competitive with specialty practices. Midwest Medical Center's administration and board felt that major redirection of the energies of Internal Medicine Group management was called for.

Organizational Changes

A number of organizational changes were implemented, one of which was MPMC's decision to bring in an individual with extensive group practice management experience. Doing so would cut the physician owner's time devoted to management issues, which in turn, it was felt, would warrant a reduction in his base salary. The physician owner would then be able to devote significantly more time to patient care, providing additional income to offset his management salary reduction. In addition, the physician owner's bonus incentive, which was related to practice acquisitions, was modified to reflect the productivity of the group. The outcome was that his incentive compensation reflected improved profitability of the group, increased volume of new patients, and expense control and reductions rather than practice acquisitions or physician recruitment.

A new computer system and conversion of the billing system became priorities. Accounts receivable were reviewed in detail, and follow-up, rebilling, and other corrective actions were taken. Additional personnel were temporarily assigned to Internal Medicine Group to accomplish these efforts.

Consultants were brought in during this process, both to provide guidance in implementing systems to correct the operational problems at Internal Medicine Group and to address the changes in the physician owner's compensation. A full report was made to the board, and realistic financial expectations were established.

Financial Performance

Internal Medicine Group has experienced significant operating losses each year since its opening in 1989. In addition to the investment of $500,000 in building and equipment expenses, significant losses from practice operations have been observed since its opening. These operating losses are primarily attributable to the low productivity of the senior physicians.

In 1992 the physician productivity was one-third below national standards for internists in group practices. (See table 6-1.) Compounding this problem, reimbursement cutbacks from Medicare and third-party payers reduced the positive financial impact of increased volume in 1993.

Billing and collection performance improved dramatically with installation of the new computer systems and guidance of the new administrator. Accounts receivable were reduced to just over 60 days, thanks to the improved accuracy of patient billing information, collections at time of service, prompt and correct filing of insurance claims, and appropriate collection efforts.

Expenses, though in actual dollars not far out of line from comparable group practices, were high relative to revenue at Internal Medicine Group. (See table 6-2.) Depreciation and interest are higher due to investment in the furnishings, equipment, renovations, and practice purchases in developing a group practice in a new facility. Nonphysician staffing levels are within industry standards, but the pay levels of employees with seniority in the practices purchased exceed average group practice salaries.

Continued efforts to maximize economies of scale of a large group are beginning to show results. This effort is supplemented by the retirements of several physicians and the acceptance of group practice operations by new physician recruits. Staff turnover has also resulted in a core group of employees whose salary level is more in line with their job responsibilities and who are better oriented to a group mentality.

Despite operating losses, the maintenance of Internal Medicine Group admissions to the hospital has been successful and offsets Internal Medicine Group losses fivefold. Although the MHM board expectation continues to be the profitable operation of Internal Medicine Group, board members recognize the overall benefit to MMC in creating

Table 6-1. Comparison of Productivity between Internal Medicine Group and MGMA Data

	Internal Medicine Group Collections per Physician	MGMA Averages[a]
1990	$144,646	$332,300
1991	160,626	342,520
1992	195,884	N/A

[a]Median reported figures from 43 internal medicine groups.

Source: Medical Group Management Association Cost Survey: 1992 Report Based on 1991 Data. Englewood, CO: MGMA, Aug. 1992, pp. 44–49.

Table 6-2. Internal Medicine Group Expenses Compared to Industry Averages

	MGMA Averages[a]		Internal Medicine Group (1991)		Internal Medicine Group (1992)	
	Dollars	%	Dollars	%	Dollars	%
Collections						
Total	N/A		$2,094,418		$2,546,488	
FTE physicians	N/A		13.5		13.0	
Collections per physician	$342,520		$ 155,142		$ 195,884	
Nonphysician Expenses (per Physician)						
Nonphysician salary and benefits	$ 84,439	24.7	$ 51,150	33.0	$ 60,724	31.0
Supplies and service	$ 41,151	12.0	$ 18,741	12.1	$ 28,246	14.4
Building occupancy expense	$ 19,362	5.7	$ 22,340	14.4	$ 24,564	12.5
Equipment and depreciation	$ 3,526	1.0	$ 8,905	5.7	$ 11,381	5.8
Insurance	$ 5,017	1.5	$ 2,824	1.8	$ 4,897	2.5
Interest	$ 1,785	0.5	$ 10,581	6.8	$ 0	0.0
Other	$ 11,267	3.3	$ 12,473	8.0	$ 10,617	5.4
Total Expenses	$166,547	48.6	$127,014	81.9	$140,429	71.7

[a]Median reported figures from 43 internal medicine groups.

Source: Medical Group Management Association Cost Survey: 1992 Report Based on 1991 Data. Englewood, CO: MGMA, Aug. 1992, pp. 44–49.

and maintaining a growing primary care network in the new health care paradigm. The clinic manager reports regularly to the board, and the results of operational improvements are monitored by the board.

Operations

Throughout 1993 the physician owner worked with group physicians to bring patient volume up to an acceptable level and maximize the efficient utilization of resources. He remains involved in operations but has turned over management concerns to the new clinic manager. His leadership has been redirected toward physician activity so as to create a truly effective group practice, manage resources in the delivery of care, and increase patient volume. Management has designed and implemented a new physician compensation system that better aligns physician incentives to manage expenses as well as reward them for higher productivity.

Lessons Learned

From an administrative standpoint, MMC has survived a tough learning process to gain an understanding of medical practice management. There is clear recognition among hospital leaders that the failure to bring in an experienced group practice manager compromised the process from the start. However, there is also conviction that the gain in understanding of physician practice operations will serve the hospital well as integration continues between the hospital and its total medical staff.

From the perspective of the medical staff, acceptance of the development of Internal Medicine Group has been attained. In part this is due to its centralized location and growth through the assimilation of existing practices, which has posed no significant threat to other primary care providers on the medical staff. Resistance from specialists to expanding Internal Medicine Group into a multispecialty group continues, but educational efforts and the realities of a changing reimbursement environment are penetrating the resistance.

Achievement of the initial goal of consolidating the large number of retiring physician practices from MMC's internal medicine department into a primary care group practice was outstanding. Significant problems were addressed throughout implementation of the group practice.

Midwest Medical Center reviewed the critical success factors identified during planning stages as the focus for practice implementation. These factors were reevaluated and are now identified as follows:

- A practice purchase package related to actual performance of existing practices
- Selection of a physician leader with proven skills in assimilating physicians into the management process
- Administrative management with strong group practice experience
- Emphasis on the building of practices for young physicians
- Shared risk among physicians with regard to the bottom line for group practice operations
- Contractual expectation of physician retirement dates
- Creation of a group practice mentality among physicians joining the group

The initial goals in developing the Internal Medicine Group, which were to assist retiring physicians and develop a large primary care group, have been achieved through the transition of a large number of primary care practices into an MMC-supported group. With the retirement of several senior physicians, Internal Medicine Group stands positioned to recruit younger primary care physicians whose productivity levels should match the committed resources. The process of creating, implementing, and maintaining management systems for this group practice provided the foundation for an expanded MSO for the center and its medical staff. Planning has begun in the effort to expand the integrated delivery system at MMC to meet the challenges of a new health care delivery paradigm.

☐ Future Outlook

The group practice management expertise and resources developed at Internal Medicine Group have become key elements for physician integration at MMC. It is anticipated that the nonclinical MSO services of the group practice will be relocated to less-expensive space where they can be expanded and provided to other practices. The group itself will probably add other specialties, initially in primary care fields (family medicine, pediatrics) and ultimately include subspecialties and surgical specialties. Efforts are under way to restructure the Internal Medicine Group from an independent corporation to a practice owned by MMC, with the physicians employed by MMC. This restructuring, which is possible due to changes in the state's corporate practice of medicine laws, is felt to be the most appropriate structure for the future integrated system.

Chapter 7

The Mercy Medical Foundation

*Vince Schmitz, Senior Vice-President and Chief Financial Officer,
Mercy Healthcare Sacramento, Sacramento, CA,
and Ronald C. Dobler, Former Executive Director, Mercy Medical
Foundation, Sacramento, CA*

☐ Executive Summary: Key Elements of the Affiliation

- *Organizational structure:* A hospital system–sponsored foundation model was created with the tax-exempt nonprofit foundation owning and operating a group practice and its assets. The foundation contracts with a freestanding physician's group (professional corporation) for professional services.
- *Hospital goals:* The system had identified a strategic need to develop an integrated network including physician practices in order to compete effectively for contracts in a reimbursement market dominated by capitation and risk sharing.
- *Physician needs and goals:* The medical group was experiencing financial difficulties due to its investment in a new clinic facility, as well as physician turnover. In addition, reduced reimbursement under fee-for-service managed care contracts and increased capitated reimbursement from insurance carriers were shrinking clinic revenues. Physicians in the group recognized the strategic need to affiliate with a hospital in order to compete effectively in a challenging health care environment. Nonclinic physicians on the medical staff were concerned that an affiliation would reduce support available to them through independent physician (or practice) association (IPA) structures and other activities.
- *Personal relationships:* Leaders in the system and the clinic had developed good personal relationships through their participation in a joint contract with a health maintenance organization. The clinic investigated affiliation with an entrepreneurial group and concluded that an affiliation with the system would provide maximum benefits. Nonclinic physician staff members, particularly those involved in an IPA, objected to an affiliation, but the hospital system continued its pursuit despite these objections.
- *Health care reform and managed care:* The high penetration of capitated managed care products in the Sacramento market was a key motivator for creating a hospital–group practice affiliation.
- *Market and competitor activities:* Strong competition from the integrated Kaiser System, as well as from other hospitals and physician groups, further recommended an affiliation. The clinic recognized the need for capital not only to meet current

debt requirements but also to develop geographic penetration to compete effectively for managed care contracts.

- *Capital needs and resources:* The hospital system was very concerned over the capital requirements for purchase of the practice. This concern led to agreement with the physician group to modify practice patterns in order to maximize revenues under capitated reimbursement. Purchase included intangible and hard assets of the practice. Capital needs and start-up financing were provided through loans to the foundation from the hospital system.
- *Physician recruitment and retention:* The number of clinic physicians who provide services to the foundation has grown through the integration of existing practices as well as the recruitment of new physicians. The sale of the clinic to the foundation significantly reduced physician buy-in requirements of the practice, which also bolstered physician recruitment.
- *Legal and contracting issues:* This foundation was one of the first established by a California hospital, and significant legal review was needed. Clinic compensation for professional services was reviewed closely to ensure compliance with regulations and laws related to private inurement and Medicare fraud and abuse. The major contractual issue was compensation for physician services.

☐ Introduction

By the late 1980s, both Mercy Healthcare Sacramento (the System), a three-hospital system, and the 62-physician Medical Clinic of Sacramento (the Clinic) had experience in capitated managed care products and were aware of the importance of an integrated health care delivery system where hospitals and physicians shared risk in order to survive in a market dominated by capitated reimbursement. This basic understanding has guided both organizations to a successful integration between a hospital system and a large group practice.

In October 1990, the System purchased the Clinic's practice and assets through a foundation created for the acquisition. The Mercy Medical Foundation (the Foundation) became one of the first hospital-sponsored foundations to own and operate a group practice in California.

The Sacramento metropolitan area has a population of 1.5 million. The city's economy was strong at the time of the integration initiative, with an annual population growth rate in excess of 2 percent and low unemployment rates. Employment was dominated by the state and federal government. Recent closure of military bases and cutbacks in state government employment have since slowed the economy and population growth, and unemployment is on the rise.

Managed Care

Managed care was introduced to the Sacramento market in the 1960s, and by the mid-1980s more than 50 percent of the population was insured through managed care products. The Kaiser System controlled the majority of the capitated market through its closed system of hospitals and physician employees and was able to offer health care buyers a well-developed, integrated, capitated delivery system. Other hospitals and practices had entered into managed care contracts but did not provide a truly integrated system of risk sharing, utilization management, and cost control mechanisms. Contracts were based on traditional fee-for-service and per diem agreements. Both physicians and hospitals were experiencing significantly reduced revenues and losses under these managed care contracts and were seeking risk-sharing arrangements where reduced costs and utilization controls could enhance the bottom line through capitated reimbursement.

Hospitals

Inpatient services in Sacramento are dominated by four multihospital systems. Kaiser Permanente controls one-third of the market; the Sutter System and Mercy Healthcare Sacramento control approximately one-quarter each; and the University of California System controls the balance.

Mercy Healthcare Sacramento has operated hospitals in the Sacramento area since 1896. By the mid-1980s it operated three local hospitals. In the past five years, it has purchased a fourth hospital and affiliated with a fifth in the area. The development of a multihospital system is the result of a strategic planning process begun in the mid-1980s that identified a shifting population base and the need to reduce and consolidate hospital facilities and services based on utilization projections.

The System has consolidated board functions, financial management, purchasing, risk management, and billings for its member hospitals into the System offices and is implementing a centralized data-processing system. In addition, four options for integration of patient services are being pursued:

1. *Centralization:* Services or staff functions provided at one location, which serves the entire system (for example, neonatal intensive care)
2. *Consolidation:* Services provided at multiple sites, but under centralized system management and staff (for example, inpatient rehabilitation)
3. *Standardization:* Services provided on a decentralized basis, but utilizing standard procedural guidelines developed for the System
4. *Decentralization:* Services delivered independently and utilizing procedural guidelines developed at more than one site

Integration among the System member hospitals continues under the guidance of the common board and has already generated significant operational savings among the hospitals.

Mercy System/Medical Staff Affiliation Efforts

Internally, the System has been successful in developing and expanding services through strong physician relations. Service line development, such as heart surgery and rehabilitation, was achieved through collaboration with key specialty physicians. Physicians are supported in numerous ways, including paid positions of leadership in the hospital operations, recruiting assistance to specialty practices, joint venturing of ancillary services, and other activities.

The System also assisted its medical staff in developing IPAs at its member hospitals in the mid-1980s. These organizations were specialty dominated and sought to maximize reimbursement levels and patient volume for the member physicians through contracting with managed care insurance companies. These contracts were based on negotiated fee-for-service reimbursement to the physician and per diem reimbursement for hospital care. By 1989 the IPAs had grown to 600 physicians and were merged into one IPA, with 25,000 lives covered under managed care contracts.

In 1985 the System acquired the franchise to provide services in the Sacramento area from a large, statewide capitated HMO. Because the IPAs were not fully developed at that time, physician services were contracted by the System through individual contracts. The System assumed full risk for this contract, as physicians were reimbursed under a negotiated fee-for-service arrangement from the capitated dollars received by the System.

In addition, the System established a management services organization (MSO) in 1985 called The Mercy Alliance. This entity was called a group practice without walls (GPWW) despite the independence of the physician practices. Through a for-profit subsidiary, the System purchased existing practices' hard assets and accounts receivables, set up practices for new physicians, and provided centralized management and operating services for the GPWW such as billing, staffing, accounting, and administrative supervision. The physicians purchased shares in the GPWW for a minimal amount (under $5,000) and created a board to deal with the hospital management company contract. Each practice operated independently, with common management services but no centralized governance or operating policies. Each practice received its own revenues, from which the practice paid the GPWW for the management services it provided and distributed the remaining dollars to its physicians.

Mercy System Financial Concerns

The System experienced operating losses in its inpatient facilities, which, coupled with losses from these medical staff affiliation efforts, created a $20 million deficit for the System in 1987. The HMO was poorly underwritten and suffered operating losses of approximately $5 million due to the inappropriate incentives and lack of risk sharing in the discounted fee-for-service reimbursement structure with physicians. In addition, the program failed to implement adequate utilization control mechanisms on the services rendered to a capitated population. The cost of purchasing practice assets and establishing a centralized medical practice operating system and a lack of expense controls caused The Mercy Alliance GPWW to experience losses of $5 million in 1987.

In 1987, the System discontinued its rights to the HMO franchise (although the System did continue as a contracted inpatient provider to that HMO) and dissolved The Mercy Alliance, allowing physicians to purchase back their practice assets from the GPWW. In 1988 and 1989, continued consolidation of services among the hospitals and termination of the HMO contract and GPWW reduced operating expenses, and the System showed small profits in both of these years.

Medical Clinic of Sacramento

The majority of physicians in the Sacramento area operated in small group or solo practices in the early 1980s. The Medical Clinic of Sacramento was formed in 1949 through the merger of several existing practices. The Clinic had physicians located in a central office and several smaller office sites in close proximity to the central office in downtown Sacramento. It functioned as an integrated group practice in terms of operating systems, income distribution, resource sharing, and centralized management. In 1987 the group expanded, both in number of physicians and patient volume, mandating a move into a new office building under a long-term lease. For the first time the group operated in a central facility as a multispecialty group practice. By 1990 it had grown to 62 physicians representing 14 specialties and had developed several satellite locations outside downtown Sacramento to provide accessibility to a growing patient base.

Clinic Financial Concerns

The Clinic faced significant financial concerns in the late 1980s. The long-term lease on the new building increased the cost of occupancy for the group from 6 to 12 percent of its revenues. The new building was to be constructed by a local developer, who planned to obtain financing for the facility based on a long-term lease with the group. The original plan did not require personal guarantees from the individual physicians of the Clinic. However, the developer was unable to complete the project as planned and personal guarantees related to the long-term lease were required from the physicians to complete the building as well as to equip and furnish the facility. Establishment of the satellite locations compounded this need for capital financing.

Additionally, the group did not achieve its budgeted revenue levels in 1986 through 1988, creating significant operating losses. Revenues had been projected too optimistically in the increasingly competitive Sacramento environment. A number of physicians left the group during this period due to concerns over the personal guarantees required on the Clinic loans, as well as the poor revenue performance. This further reduced revenues. Debt was incurred to offset the operating deficits. A buy-in requirement of more than $40,000 was imposed on new physicians joining the Clinic, up from the historic level of $20,000.

The buy-in proved to be an insurmountable obstacle in the Clinic's recruiting efforts; the competing Kaiser organization was able to guarantee physicians a large income with no buy-in. The Clinic, unable to recruit new physicians or replacements for the physicians who had left, found itself losing market share.

Mercy System–Medical Clinic Relationship

During the first 30 years of its existence, the Clinic had admitted the majority of its inpatients to the Sutter Health System hospitals. Clinic leaders had determined in the early 1980s that inpatient admissions should be made to other hospitals in order for the group to maintain active privileges in several hospital systems and position itself to participate in managed care contracts exclusive to more than one hospital system.

HMO Contract
In 1985 the Clinic entered a capitated contract for physician services with Take Care HMO and approached Mercy Healthcare Sacramento to accept the hospital contract offered by Take Care. This step for stronger association with the Mercy System was a result of the Clinic's strategy to affiliate with other hospitals as well as unsuccessful negotiations between Take Care and the Sutter System. As a result, Mercy contracted with this HMO in 1985.

Because of California insurance regulations, HMO contracts with the Clinic and the hospital were separate and independent. A "global" capitated rate, including physician and hospital services, could not be offered in California by an HMO. However, because both entities were in risk-sharing agreements involving the same population, ongoing communication between the System and Clinic leadership was quickly established through this relationship.

Despite its increasing participation in capitated reimbursement contracts, the Clinic continued to operate under a fee-for-service mentality. Tightening financial pressures at the Clinic—a result of increased expense and reduced revenues—created traditional reactions from the physicians: cut costs, increase services, and maximize billings. Minimal effort or investment was put into the utilization management of capitated patients. Information systems did not provide adequate clinical or financial analysis of the practice, physicians did not avail themselves of appropriate utilization review or cost reduction tools, and management resources were devoted to "tightening the belt" rather than marketing, negotiating, and monitoring contracts.

Building Costs
As costs of the Clinic's relocation to a consolidated facility escalated, the System became concerned as a result of the HMO arrangement with the Clinic. Therefore the System provided financial support to the developer in order to relieve some of the debt burden on the Clinic. Banks had been unwilling to fund the debt based on the individual physician guarantees alone, especially as the group lost physicians and experienced decreasing revenues.

Practice Sale Discussions
In 1988 the Clinic entered discussions with PhyCor, a Nashville, Tennessee–based for-profit entity that purchases group practice assets and works with group physicians (as an independent professional corporation) in operating the practice. Negotiations over the sale of the Clinic to PhyCor followed. Ultimately, the Clinic decided that the opportunities with this organization were not in its best interests. The physicians had concerns over absentee ownership of their practice assets and loss of control of the

management of their practice to outsiders. Also, PhyCor did not offer a purchase price that would both retire the Clinic debt and provide significant payment for the practice to the physicians. The Clinic physicians felt that the practice would be of more value and experience the best success in an affiliation with a local health care organization. The PhyCor offer was rejected despite concern over the Clinic's future financial picture.

☐ Motivations for Affiliations

This section briefly delineates the circumstances that drove the Mercy System toward integration with a physician group. Motivations from both perspectives—those of the System and those of the Clinic physicians—are identified.

Hospital Motivations

Catholic Healthcare West (CHW), the parent company of Mercy Healthcare Sacramento, operates in three states and owns 17 hospitals. Many CHW hospitals are in locations with significant capitated insurance products and, like the Mercy System, had experienced financial losses under risk-sharing arrangements. In studying the reasons for poor success in managed care contract results among member hospitals, CHW determined that a structure that integrated physician practices with hospital operations was the answer. Comparing its strategies to the Kaiser integrated system approach, which competed in most CHW hospital markets, dramatically supported this conclusion. By the late 1980s, this conclusion had been incorporated into a strategy for CHW hospitals to establish viable structures. For its California hospitals, CHW recommended a foundation model for integration, because of the state's corporate practice of medicine regulations.

Geographically, the Mercy System was in an excellent position to provide care to the population of Sacramento. The three hospitals currently in the network provided accessible inpatient care to most of the city's population. However, their inadequate experience under capitated contracting and inability to develop physician risk-sharing arrangements reinforced CHW's conclusion that full integration was needed.

Therefore the System sought partnership with a physician group by means of which the System and physicians would have mutual financial goals for implementing the needed systems and clinical practice changes to effect a successful risk-sharing contract. Because of the failures with earlier joint contracting efforts, the System's leaders recognized that without full physician commitment, cost savings would not be sufficient to provide care under capitated contracts.

Physician Motivations

Clinic physicians also recognized their need for an integrated delivery system through the Clinic's experience with managed care. Decreasing physician revenues in a capitated environment, even in a large group practice situation, motivated the Clinic to seek a true risk-sharing situation with an organization providing inpatient and ancillary services. In addition, the financial problems created by the new building and recruitment limitations created a need for the Clinic to find a source of capital.

Initiation of Affiliation Discussions

Through involvement in funding for the Clinic building and the long-term HMO agreement, System financial personnel had begun meeting regularly with the Clinic administration. The System was able to provide positive input into the building design and construction and the Clinic operations in the new facility. Between 1985 and 1988, the Clinic and the System developed a relationship based on mutual trust. Admissions of

Clinic patients to the Mercy System continued to increase. Planning discussions held between leaders of both parties disclosed mutual motivations for an affiliation.

□ Planning

The planning process for formal affiliation between the Clinic and Mercy System occurred over a 12-month period beginning in 1989. The mutual benefits of an affiliation were recognized by the leadership of both organizations, but they decided to keep the planning process confidential until a structure was identified that could address the major issues they anticipated from their organizations, as detailed in the following sections. The planning group, consisting of the System's senior vice-president of finance, its senior vice-president of strategic planning, and the Clinic administrator, agreed on the key issues to be resolved by each organization.

The fact that the planning group was small and made up of individuals with business backgrounds facilitated the process. The Clinic's president and executive committee and the System's president and board were kept apprised of planning activities and guided their representatives throughout the process.

Hospital Issues

The planning group anticipated that the System would be concerned over three key issues: cost, the medical staff's response to a proposed affiliation, and the Clinic's commitment to risk sharing. The concern over cost had to do with the capital investment required to acquire the Clinic. Failure of the GPWW several years earlier had been attributed in part to the purchase price for practice assets demanded by the physicians joining the GPWW.

As for how the medical staff would respond, the fact that the affiliation effort would affect only a small percentage of the 1,000-member medical staff was identified as a key issue. Despite acceptance of the strategy to develop an integrated system, there was concern that other medical staff members would react negatively to a System–Clinic affiliation.

The System representatives expressed concern over the Clinic's commitment to share risk under a capitated contract and to implement the changes needed in practice patterns and operations for success in a capitated environment. The Clinic received 75 percent of its revenues through fee-for-service reimbursement, and individual physician compensation was based on procedure productivity. Continuation of this approach would make physician practice incentives counterproductive to success under capitated reimbursement.

Clinic Issues

The Clinic was concerned with one overriding issue—its potential loss of identity and autonomy through assimilation into the System. The physicians had rejected earlier affiliations based on this potential loss of control, specifically control of decisions on the addition or removal of physicians from the group, physician income from the practice, medical decisions and protocols, and managed care contract review and selection.

This concern was offset by the Clinic's need to eliminate the debt and ensure adequate capital to support operating needs including expansion and recruitment. The physicians realized that Clinic buy-in requirements restricted their ability to attract new physicians or invest in further expansion of facilities or services needed to provide care to populations under managed care contracts. Further, the physicians were uncomfortable with individual guarantees on Clinic debt required of each physician.

Affiliation Structure

It had been agreed that the Clinic needed to sell its assets, relieve its debt burden, and have access to capital in order to survive and grow. The planning group determined that a foundation model provided a mechanism for the System to finance the purchase and maintain physicians' input into practice operations and strategies. Equally important was the fact that this structure provided physician control over medical decisions such as quality of care, physician membership, clinical protocols, role of nonphysician staff in providing services, and so forth. The planning group consulted leaders of both organizations as the process continued, and a consultant was hired to develop a business plan for the Clinic's purchase.

In the 1970s California had passed enabling legislation for the creation of foundations to operate medical practices. This legislation designated criteria for tax-exempt foundations to meet in order to comply with licensure requirements under the state's corporate practice of medicine laws. The legislation, passed on behalf of private group practices, had not been applied to a hospital-owned foundation practice at the time planning was under way for the System's purchase of the Clinic assets using a foundation model. Some basic conditions for the development of a foundation under California regulations included the following:

- Creation of a 501(c)(3) corporation to operate the practice, with requirements to provide medical services to the community at large
- A minimum of 40 physicians representing 10 specialists, at least 66 percent of whom practice full-time
- Pursuit of medical research and health education activities

These requirements could be met through establishment of a new foundation to purchase the Clinic assets and contract with the physician group for professional services. Medical research and health education activities were incorporated into plans for the foundation prototype.

Through the foundation model, the hospital was able to provide financing for the purchase of Clinic assets, medical records, consideration for goodwill, and the assumption of debts from the group. Physicians were able to remain in a separate professional corporation, retaining control over their group and its practice, and to receive an agreed-on percentage of professional revenue. Physicians would be responsible for professional considerations and the medical care delivered in the foundation and for physician recruitment. Physician income distributions would be determined in this professional corporation.

It was felt that this structure represented a true partnership. The Mercy Medical Foundation would assume administrative responsibilities for the practice and enhance the practice with the System's management and operational resources while the Clinic retained control over the professional activities. Figure 7-1 reflects the organizational structure of the System, including the Foundation.

Announcement of the Plan

The plan to purchase the Clinic was formally presented to the board of directors of Mercy Healthcare Sacramento. As anticipated, the board was concerned with this strategy and questioned the financial return to the System from a large capital investment. The board sought the advice of an independent consulting group working with the System on the development and implementation of a strategic plan.

Based on research of the Sacramento market, activities of competitor hospital systems, and insurance company programs, as well as current operations of the System and Clinic, the consultants concluded that developing a foundation to purchase Clinic assets was a sound strategy. Catholic Healthcare West's experience in other markets was also reviewed, and several locations were visited where integrated systems were competing successfully with nonintegrated hospitals and medical groups. Other foundations already established by medical practices in California were studied.

The System also had concerns about the Clinic's ability to modify its compensation incentives and practice patterns to operate in a capitated reimbursement environment. These concerns were alleviated by the experience with the long-term Take Care HMO contract. Clinic leadership could demonstrate improved utilization for the enrollees of that contract. In addition, the income distribution of the Clinic had been modified to include a larger percentage of each physician's income coming from the overall financial results of the Clinic (equal distribution) rather than from each physician's actual practice productivity.

The proposal to create a structure that integrated the hospitals and physicians in a risk-sharing structure was endorsed by the consultants and accepted by the board. The

Figure 7-1. Mercy Medical Foundation Organizational Chart

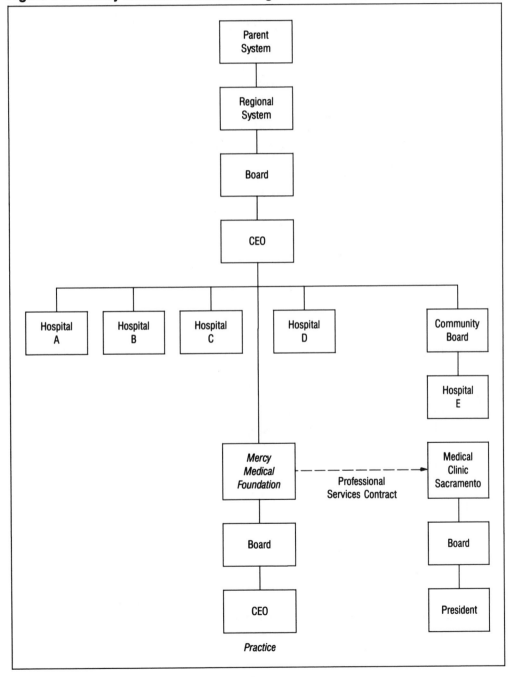

purchase of the Clinic was accepted as the initial step in this direction, and a letter of intent to purchase was drafted and presented to the Clinic. The letter of intent included an agreement that the Clinic would not enter discussions with any other entity during the period of negotiation with the System.

Presentation of the plan for the sale of the Clinic's assets to a System-sponsored foundation was accepted by Clinic physicians as an appropriate strategy, but it did raise issues of physician control and autonomy in the practice. Despite the level of trust between the Clinic and System leadership, the physicians feared that their practice patterns would be dictated by the System. Following discussion of the letter of intent, it was determined that significant education and communication with physicians would be required to overcome these concerns.

Medical Staff Reaction

The announcement of plans to purchase the Clinic's assets brought an outcry from the System's medical staff and the IPA specifically. In 1989 IPA leaders demanded an emergency meeting with the hospital administrators that was attended by more than 200 physicians.

The System presented its strategy for dealing with the changing environment, including medical staff affiliation activities. The variety of efforts implemented by the System were reviewed, such as development of a multihospital system to gain efficiencies and geographic coverage, as well as multiple approaches to dealing with physicians. The development and support of the IPA, the GPWW, work with specialty departments, recruitment activities, and the Clinic purchase were some of the topics discussed. The hospital related the experience from the previous HMO arrangements with physicians and defined the need for a strong integration with the medical staff. Emphasis was placed on the fact that the Clinic purchase was only part of an overall strategy for working with the medical staff.

The physicians on the medical staff were not placated but did not protest the plan formally. The negotiations and implementation of the Clinic purchase took the next nine months for completion, and during this period much of the medical staff concern dissipated. The IPAs continued to contract with managed care companies, and, two years later, the System assisted in an affiliation between their IPA and a San Francisco IPA, greatly enhancing its contracting appeal and benefit to the medical staff membership in the IPA.

☐ Negotiations

The Clinic and System pursued the development of a foundation model and purchase of Clinic assets despite medical staff objections. The consultants continued to develop a business plan, and the System's legal staff began review and documentation for the creation of a foundation. The planning team was assigned to complete the negotiations.

System Issues

The board of directors was most concerned about the capital investment required to purchase the Clinic. Board members did not want to jeopardize the System's financial situation in a way similar to the earlier GPWW effort. A foundation model offered the opportunity for tax-exempt financing, but after review it was determined that the System would provide the initial financing in the form of loans to the Mercy Medical Foundation. The business plan was carefully reviewed to ensure that the Foundation's revenues could absorb existing debt as well as the costs of purchase and merger over a five-year period. The business plan identified significant opportunity for the Foundation to contract with managed care plans to increase revenues. Expansion of the group would reduce the need to contract for physician services outside the Foundation. The System felt the physicians should assume risk for capitated contracts and profitable operations of the Foundation. The payment for professional services to the Clinic would need to be structured in a way that would incorporate these elements and motivate the physicians to control utilization and costs.

Clinic Issues

The most significant issue for physicians was that the Foundation operate autonomously from hospitals in the System, with physicians providing input on practice strategies and operations. The foundation model provided the desired physician control in professional areas through maintenance of the group as a freestanding professional corporation, contracted by the Mercy Medical Foundation for professional services. The professional corporation would have its own board made up of physician owners who would make decisions on physician addition or removal, income distribution among physicians, utilization improvements, quality of care, and so forth.

The Foundation would be owned by the System as a subsidiary corporation, equal in status with the hospital members, and would have its own mission statement and board of directors. The Clinic board would advise the Foundation under its contract to provide professional services and through representation on the Foundation board.

To qualify for tax-exempt financing (bonds) under California regulations, no more than 20 percent of the Clinic physicians could be members of the Foundation board. The Clinic felt that physician and System representation on the board should be equal. It was determined that the Foundation's board would have the following membership:

- President of the Clinic (elected by the physicians)
- CEO of the System
- Three representatives from the community who were unaffiliated with the Clinic or the System

The Foundation would own the practice and assets, and all nonphysician employees would work for the Foundation. All negotiations with managed care entities would be conducted by the Foundation, but the Clinic would retain veto power over contracts.

Clinic Compensation

The Clinic receives a negotiated percentage of Foundation revenues as compensation for professional services. This percentage is based on historical clinic overhead costs, fair market reimbursement for professional services, and projected operating results of the Foundation.

The initial level for Clinic reimbursement for professional services was set at approximately 50 percent of revenues and is subject to renegotiation every two years under the contract. Actual financial results of the Foundation's activities will become the dominant factor in future reimbursement to the Clinic for professional services.

Clinic Purchase

It was determined that the Foundation would purchase the Clinic's hard assets at fair market value. The valuation process included consideration for the Foundation's assumption of the remaining debt incurred by the Clinic in furnishing and equipping its new facility.

Accounts receivable of the Clinic remained with the professional corporation. For a nominal fee the Foundation would provide collection services on these existing accounts receivable. The Foundation would provide advances on future revenues to the professional corporation to fund the ongoing compensation of its physicians.

The System further agreed to purchase the practice goodwill. The basis for valuation of goodwill was determined by an independent appraisal.

The professional corporation would be a manpower entity only. That is, it would own no assets, and all of its revenues would flow through the agreement with the Foundation. Physicians recruited into the professional corporation would have a minimal buy-in requirement for stock, based on the value of the ongoing revenue flow from the Foundation. Patient admissions from the Foundation were not restricted to System hospitals, and Clinic physicians maintain privileges at other hospitals. The basis for the amount of payment for goodwill was the projected revenues of the practice under the Foundation. Individual Clinic physicians recognized that the ultimate benefit of this affiliation was not in the purchase payment, but in the ongoing strength of the Foundation in generating revenues.

☐ Implementation and Outcomes

Implementation of the foundation model has been successful. The five-year process of building trust through managed care contracts, financing the new building facility, planning and negotiating the affiliation structure, and addressing the concerns of Clinic physicians and the System board and administration led to a smooth transition to the new structure. Clinic management and operations were not displaced, and the Clinic was able to schedule stages in the transition and adapt its systems in an orderly manner. Success to date can also be attributed to ongoing efforts to increase the level of planning and management expertise of both the physicians and Foundation management staff. This has been accomplished through educational efforts and shared control of the Foundation from board participation, operational responsibilities, and committee composition involving both physicians and management representatives.

Clinic Growth

During the first 36 months following the Foundation's establishment, the Clinic grew from 62 to 117 physicians through new physician recruitment and integration of other practices. Successful recruitment eliminated physician candidate concerns about the financial viability of the practice that existed for the Clinic. Buy-in was reduced from $40,000 to $5,000 and Foundation revenues grew from $20 million in the first nine months following the purchase of the Clinic to a projected $50 million for the 1994 fiscal year. (See figure 7-2.) Physician income has stabilized under the agreement with the Foundation,

Figure 7-2. Mercy Medical Foundation Revenues

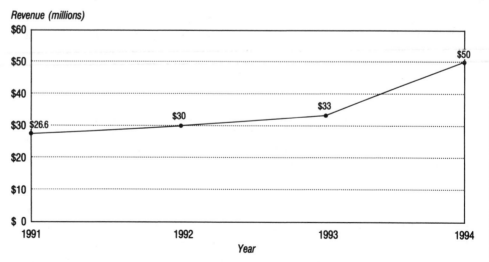

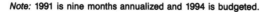 *Note:* 1991 is nine months annualized and 1994 is budgeted.

and physician candidates are presented a practice opportunity geared to survival, stability, and success under a changing reimbursement environment.

Managed Care Contracting

With the closing of the transaction, the Foundation assumed the two capitated contracts that the Clinic had entered. In the first 36 months, six additional contracts were negotiated, including two with Medicare. Capitated patient enrollment with the Foundation expanded from 28,000 to 56,000. Total patients served by the Foundation has grown to exceed 125,000.

Utilizing financial and managerial resources from the System, the Clinic has greatly enhanced its managed care contracting abilities through the Foundation. Physician members serve on Foundation committees involved in both marketing the Foundation to managed care entities as well as reviewing and negotiating contracts. The approach taken by the System and Clinic through the Foundation is a true partnership, with the decision making and resources for Foundation operations being provided by the most appropriate entity. Both the Clinic and the System retain veto rights over managed care contracts, and consensus must be reached before a new contract is entered.

Medical Staff Reaction

Establishment of the Foundation and purchase of the Clinic assets occurred without significant medical staff reaction, but the rapid Clinic expansion has refueled concern among the rest of the medical staff that the Foundation will grow to dominate the medical staff. This issue came to a head in August 1993 with the Foundation's purchase of a nine-physician primary care practice.

Again, an emergency meeting was called by the medical staff, with over 400 physicians attending. The System reinforced its message delivered at the earlier meeting, outlining its overall strategy and the Foundation's role in creating an integrated system.

The medical staff was still dissatisfied, and there was talk of boycotting the System. It is difficult to assess retroactively whether more communication with the medical staff during the planning process might have diffused their concerns. The System continues to offer alternative programs for its medical staff and is committed to moving forward with the Foundation.

Physician Risk Sharing

One of the most significant results from creation of the Foundation has been the acceptance and commitment of the group to risk sharing. Capitated contracts have grown and 80 percent of the Foundation's revenue now comes through capitated reimbursement. With the input of System resources in terms of information systems and management, the Foundation is leading the development of the utilization review process for the entire System.

The Clinic has established two HMO director positions, one a primary care physician and the other a surgical specialist. They are responsible for utilization control and contract compliance. Inpatient days for commercial HMO populations have been reduced to 133 per 1,000 patients, and 1,100 inpatient days per 1,000 Medicare patients have been accomplished through utilization review activities. These inpatient days are well below historical length of stay for the System and for national utilization rates.

Another example of the success of the new affiliation in dealing with capitated reimbursement was savings in excess of $23,000 on the prescription risk pool under a capitated contract. Historically, losses had been incurred in reimbursement for prescription activities. Efforts in educating physicians on the use of generic drugs and protocols for prescription activities affected this significant turnaround in the first 18 months.

Physician Compensation

Physicians have agreed to modify their compensation basis with the Clinic. Traditionally, physician productivity was the major basis on which compensation was paid. Effective January 1994, physicians are paid a salary based on historical compensation and fair market specialty compensation, with a bonus if additional dollars are available, distributed to physicians based on the following factors:

- Citizenship within the group; that is, compliance with group goals
- Utilization management
- Qualitative measures of satisfactory patient service (patient complaints and surveys, for example)
- Primary responsibility for capitated enrollees
- Productivity in that portion of practice revenues generated through fee-for-service reimbursement

These changes represent a true cultural evolution for the Clinic.

☐ Future Outlook

Mercy Healthcare Sacramento will continue its efforts to develop an integrated health care system to serve the city's population. The following list represents some specific goals and directions.

- *Growth and expansion:* Continued expansion of the Foundation through growth of patient volume under managed care contracts and the addition of physicians through recruitment and incorporation of existing practices. The Foundation currently practices out of 19 locations as the result of practice integration. Plans are under way to consolidate these sites into 10 sites strategically located geographically throughout the Sacramento area. This effort includes plans for a new 52,000-square-foot outpatient facility in northern Sacramento.
- *Information systems:* Plans are under way to upgrade the Foundation's information system so as to deal with the increasing volume and address the information needs that arise from practicing in a capitated environment. The Foundation's information system will be integrated with the one being implemented at the inpatient facilities to provide complete utilization and cost data.
- *Physician leadership:* The partnership with the Clinic physicians through the Foundation and the recognition of the need for strong physician leadership to effect practice pattern changes are being pursued through ongoing educational efforts. For example, 10 physicians are being sponsored by the Foundation in their attainment of MBAs.
- *Relationship enhancement:* The Foundation's relationship with the medical staff throughout all System hospitals continues to be an issue. Support of the IPA activities; opportunities for medical staff to join the Foundation; and the integration of Foundation activities into utilization review, benefiting the entire medical staff, will continue.

Chapter 8

Good Samaritan Medical Foundation—Health Dimensions, Inc.

Harry Glatstein, MD, President, Good Samaritan Medical Foundation, San Jose, CA

☐ **Executive Summary: Key Elements of the Affiliation**

- *Organizational structure:* A foundation model involving a tax-exempt nonprofit organization that owns and operates a medical practice and contracts with a free-standing physician group (professional corporation) to provide professional services for the practice. The freestanding physician group has a contract with a 300-physician IPA to provide services to the foundation's patients.
- *Hospital goals:* This three-hospital system recognized a long-term need to develop an integrated organization with the physicians on its medical staff. The strategic goal was to create an organization to accept full risk-sharing contracts with insurance companies and compete effectively in its market.
- *Physician needs and goals:* Physicians in the San Jose area were experiencing reduced reimbursement for services from managed care insurance payers and facing higher expenses in adapting their practice operations to the challenging health care delivery environment, including the need to provide access to capitated patient populations outside their practices' traditional service area. Two group practices on the hospital's medical staff were actively pursuing affiliation partners (hospitals, other physician groups, and private investors) to meet their short-term needs for capital and to address their strategic goal of developing an integrated system to deal with risk-sharing contracts. Solo practitioners on the medical staff had formed a number of PPOs and IPAs to deal with insurance contracting.
- *Personal relationships:* One of the existing group practices distrusted the hospital, based on a previous joint contracting effort with a capitated insurance product. Turnover within the hospital leadership, triggered by objections of the medical staff to an affiliation with a small group practice, also delayed the planning and negotiation process while new relationships were developed. The inability of two existing group practices to identify mutually acceptable affiliation arrangements caused one of the groups to shift its hospital allegiance to other hospital systems. A good personal relationship between the leadership of the group practice and the hospital medical staff IPA led to a successful affiliation between these two physician organizations and the hospital system.

- *Health care reform and managed care:* The San Jose market was experiencing a significant shift to capitated reimbursement. Various physician contracting groups in the medical staff sought exclusive contracts with insurance companies in competition with one another. The financial pressure from risk-sharing contracts was a major factor in developing this hospital–group practice affiliation.
- *Market and competitor activities:* Members of the medical staff competed with each other for contracts, while at the same time facing significant competition from organizations such as Kaiser. Hospitals in the market also competed for physician loyalty, admissions, and joint contracting opportunities. The hospital system was in the process of closing beds and consolidating services in their inpatient facilities as a result of reduced demand, as well as trying to coordinate activities with their medical staff.
- *Capital needs and resources:* Significant capital was required for the purchase of the existing group practice. In addition, the hospital utilized several consultants in developing a proposal that was acceptable to the physician groups. Funding for the capital required by the foundation and the start-up costs of planning and implementing the affiliated practice was provided by loans from the hospital.
- *Physician recruitment and retention:* The increase in the number of physicians in the hospital-affiliated group has come primarily through the integration of existing practices. The relationships between the group practice and the IPA structured through the affiliation has caused many physicians to leave their solo practices and join the group. The growth of patient volume through the improved contracting position of the affiliated hospital–group practice has supported this physician growth and retention.
- *Legal and contracting issues:* Significant legal issues were addressed during the creation of the foundation, purchase of the existing group, and contracting with the physician group practice for professional services. In addition, the agreement between an existing group and independent IPA to provide services to the foundation was complicated.

☐ Introduction

Health Dimensions, Inc. (HDI), now called Good Samaritan Health System, is a three-hospital system located in the San Jose/Santa Clara Valley area of California. In the late 1980s, HDI faced increasing competition for patients under managed care contracting and reduced reimbursement for inpatient services. Study of these issues raised HDI's awareness of the effectiveness of integrated delivery systems in dealing with the changing health care environment, and HDI approached a large group practice on its medical staff concerning the development of an affiliation structure. Planning and negotiations expanded to include another group practice and a 280-physician-member IPA. In April 1992 the Good Samaritan Medical Foundation (the Foundation) was formed with the Good Samaritan Medical Group (GSMG), a 27-physician multispecialty group practice, and the IPA.

The Foundation grew rapidly during its first 12 months of operations. It also has played a major role in leading HDI and its medical staff to achieve the changes in health care delivery patterns required for success in a capitated environment.

☐ Background

The San Jose/Santa Clara area has a population of approximately 1.4 million. Its economy was very strong throughout the 1980s, reflecting the growth of data-processing industries located in the "Silicon Valley." More recently, the economy has stalled; growing unemployment and population declines have increased competition among health care providers for managed care contracts.

Through the mid-1980s, the Kaiser HMO and integrated hospital–physician delivery systems dominated the capitated care market in the San Jose/Santa Clara area. By 1988 Kaiser had enrolled approximately 40 percent of the population in its capitated program.

Other managed care products were predominantly discounted fee-for-service reimbursement to the physicians, based on individual practice contracts and per diem reimbursement for inpatient care. The changing economic environment was forcing a rapid transition of these managed care programs to capitated products.

Hospital

Health Dimensions, Inc., was created as a result of the merger of two large hospitals in the San Jose area. During the 1980s, two additional hospitals were acquired and ultimately closed; their beds were incorporated into existing HDI hospitals and a new hospital in the system that was built in the rural southern end of San Jose County.

By 1989 the three hospitals were consolidated into a 1,000-bed system with common management and operating resources. The system was experiencing operating losses due to the costs associated with the acquisitions and consolidations, as well as decreasing admissions and reimbursement. In addition to the two Kaiser hospitals located in the HDI market area, competition for patients included seven other hospitals.

Physicians

Medical staff at HDI included two large multispecialty physician groups. The San Jose Medical Group (SJMG) was formed in the late 1940s, and by 1989 it had grown to 65 physicians. The GSMG was formed in 1986 through combination of the practices of seven internists, four pediatricians, and two OB/GYN physicians. By 1989 the group had grown to 18 physicians. With the exception of these two multispecialty groups, physicians in the San Jose area had solo practices or small group practices.

In the mid-1980s, a physicians practice organization (PPO) was formed for the purpose of reviewing and recommending contracts for physician practices. This PPO was independent of the hospital, and approximately 50 percent of the HDI medical staff participated. The PPO did not attempt to attract capitated contracts or engage in independent risk-sharing tactics such as cost sharing, utilization review, or economic credentialing of physicians. The PPO was dominated by specialists, whose purpose was to identify and negotiate contracts with maximum fee-for-service reimbursement.

In 1986 Aetna Insurance sought to create a closed-panel, IPA-model HMO in the San Jose area. Aetna offered capitated reimbursement to primary care physicians who would function in a gatekeeper role for the contract's enrollees. Specialists were to be contracted by Aetna and reimbursed under negotiated fee arrangements. The PPO was unwilling to enter this type of contract with Aetna, and 300 physicians elected to create a new IPA structure to provide services under this contract; GSMG became a member of this IPA.

The IPA elected a board of directors, and negotiations with Aetna led to contract completion in 1987, with HDI being contracted as the inpatient provider. The IPA negotiated with Aetna for its members to be the exclusive physician providers under this contract. Aetna provided all claims processing and information system requirements for the IPA. The IPA provided credentialing for the participating physicians as well as ongoing utilization review activities through board review of practice activities and committee activities, staffed by IPA physicians.

HDI–Medical Staff Relations

Until 1988 HDI had focused its activities on the acquisition and consolidation of its hospitals. Because managed care contracts were offered to physicians and hospitals independently, HDI entered contracts with as many managed care companies as possible to support the inpatient needs of its medical staff. Because the PPO focused on maximizing the physician component in managed care contracting, the relationship between this organization and HDI was minimal. As the IPA developed its capitated relationship with Aetna, coordination between HDI and leadership of the IPA in controlling the utilization under this contract was increased.

During the 1980s HDI was dealing with integration of medical staffs from its most recent hospital acquisitions into its systemwide medical staff and was hesitant to develop formal relationships with any specific groups of physicians. Instead, HDI focused on providing services and inpatient beds under managed care contracting to all members of its medical staff. An exception to this policy was HDI's development of four satellite urgi-care centers in 1985. The system invested $6 million in the facilities and start-up operations of these urgicenters, contracting with the SJMG to provide physician coverage and management.

□ Motivations for Affiliation

Competition for and profitable performance under managed care contracts were the primary motivators for affiliation discussions between HDI and the two medical groups on its medical staff. Health Dimensions, Inc., felt an integrated system of physicians and hospitals was needed to compete with the Kaiser HMO. Purchasers of health care in the San Jose/Santa Clara area were demanding reductions in their health care expenditures. Existing managed care contracts could not compete with Kaiser in reducing the cost of health care delivery.

The administrative leadership of HDI was motivated to increase volume through managed care contracting but recognized that effective cost savings and utilization review could not be achieved without a structure through which to share risk and reward with physicians. Eventually HDI accepted a contract with an HMO involving shared risk pools for the HMO's savings on capitated premiums through physician and inpatient utilization reductions. The San Jose Medical Group contracted with this HMO to be the exclusive provider of physician care. Reimbursement was on a discounted fee-for-service basis for the SJMG physicians and on a per diem basis for HDI. By 1989 this program had 22,000 enrollees, but there were business conflicts between SJMG and HDI. As a result, HDI believed a more formal affiliation between physicians and hospitals was needed to implement risk-sharing contracting with physicians.

Concurrently, the Good Samaritan Medical Group was pursuing strategies to increase its managed care contracting volume. A conflict with the IPA under its exclusive Aetna contract had led to GSMG's dropping out of that organization. The IPA had been unwilling to subcapitate GSMG, insisting that reimbursement to the group be based on individual physician activity similar to other IPA physician members. The GSMG withdrew from the IPA and was terminated from the Aetna contract. Subsequently, GSMG entered two contracts with other managed care companies to be the exclusive physician provider to their enrollees. By 1989 approximately 15,000 lives were enrolled by GSMG through these contracts. The GSMG continued to subcontract individually with specialists and surgeons who were members of the IPA for services not available in the group.

The competition for exclusive rights as the physician providers for managed care contracts was intense. Both medical groups had significant debt as a result of facility improvement and expansion, including the recruitment of new physicians. Capital investment in providing expanded geographic coverage and the development of management and information systems to control utilization and costs were clear needs for both groups to help them gain an advantage in winning contracts from managed care products.

☐ Planning

Planning efforts for an affiliation with physicians began within HDI. A consultant was hired, and, with input from HDI administrators, various options for development of an integrated structure were reviewed. The foundation model was identified as the most appropriate structure through which the system could incorporate existing medical groups. Key reasons were that a foundation model complied with the corporate practice of medicine laws in California and the success of the foundation model in other parts of the state.

The planning and negotiation process for development of a foundation occurred between October 1989 and June 1992. A time line for this process is presented in figure 8-1.

Initial Planning Effort between HDI and Medical Groups

In 1989 HDI began a series of meetings with SJMG concerning development of a foundation model to share risk under capitated contracts. Discussions with SJMG were initiated by HDI for the following reasons:

- SJMG was the largest group practice in the area.
- A relationship between HDI and SJMG already existed in the urgi-care centers agreement and the "risk pool" HMO contract.

Figure 8-1. Planning and Negotiation Process and Time Line

October 1989:	HDI and SJMG begin meetings to discuss development of an integrated model (foundation).
January 1990:	Good Samaritan Medical Group joins discussions.
January–July 1990:	Biweekly meetings concerning consolidation of the groups and development of the foundation.
July 1990:	Joint retreat held to discuss foundation and letter of intent. Differences between groups and concern over HDI control of Foundation cause all discussions to end.
July 1990–February 1991:	Both groups look for alternate partners. Offers to GSMG to affiliate with other hospitals, venture capital groups, and insurance companies are made but not accepted.
May 1991:	HDI makes new proposal to SJMG and GSMG to develop Foundation. SJMG is not really interested, and they pursue other hospitals in the area. GSMG reviews, discusses, and decides to go for this proposal.
May–September 1991:	Consultants brought to educate the HDI Board and GSMG physicians on changing goals and objectives in an integrated system. HDI and GSMC continue to meet on details of affiliation.
November 1991:	Letter of intent signed by HDI and GSMG. Attorneys begin work on application for Foundation.
December 1991:	Reaction of rest of HDI medical staff to letters of intent to develop a foundation very "hostile." HDI board stops continued discussions with GSMG and investigates integration of additional physicians into Foundation. HDI board selects IPA for inclusion in Foundation.
January 1992:	GSMG investigates affiliation with SJMG, but differences still exist. GSMG begins meetings with IPA. HDI administrators forced to resign due to medical staff conflict.
February 1992:	GSMG, IPA, and HDI agree on issues of governance and reserved rights for the Foundation. Valuation of GSMG completed.
March 1992:	Final legal and financial issues are discussed. IRS approval obtained as nonprofit foundation.
April 1, 1992:	Nonprofit foundation officially forms, purchases GSMG, and begins operations.
June 1992:	Managed care agreement between GSMG, IPA, and GSMF signed. First + Care sites (four) from old agreement with HDI and SJMG phased into GSMF.

- The SJMG traditionally had admitted the majority of its patients to HDI.
- The SJMG had expressed an interest in investigating an affiliation.

Planning was engineered by the senior vice-president of HDI, the president of SJMG, and the consultant. In early 1990, the GSMG was asked to join in this effort because of the need for a larger number of physicians with expanded geographic coverage in order for the Foundation to market itself effectively to managed care programs. The GSMG represented the only other multispecialty group practice in the HDI system that was doing significant managed care on an assumption of risk basis.

From the start, there were differences and distrust between the two group practices. The SJMG was a much larger group and felt that it should dominate the physician component of the Foundation. Both groups had significant debt, but SJMG had far more assets. Retirement plans were structured differently, as were physician compensation bases; compensation was production based in SJMG and salary based in GSMG. Furthermore, the overall group cultures differed.

Planning sessions were conducted on a biweekly basis over a six-month period, and in July 1990 a retreat was held for the boards of all three organizations. The retreat was a disaster, and the differences that separated the two groups, coupled with their mutual distrust, curtailed further discussion of the potential benefits of affiliation.

In addition, neither physician group was comfortable with the approach HDI was taking to develop an integrative structure. Clearly HDI had determined that control of the affiliated practice by the hospital system was required—the proposed structure included a preponderance of HDI representatives on Foundation governing boards, operating committees, and leadership positions.

Following the retreat, a letter of intent was drawn up by HDI and rejected by both groups. The planning process came to an end.

Medical Groups Pursue Other Affiliations

Between July 1990 and May 1991, both groups' need for capital led them to seek new partners. The GSMG received offers for affiliation from other hospital systems, insurance companies, and a venture capital group that was developing a large MSO physician network. It was felt that involvement in all of these organizations would have adverse impact on the operations of the group. Not only were there control issues should the medical practice affiliate with these organizations, but an affiliation also would force the group to admit its patients to another hospital. Historically GSMG had used HDI, and the prospect of using other hospitals made the group's physicians uncomfortable. The SJMG also pursued opportunities for financial support or affiliation with other organizations but was unable to identify a relationship in which it could maintain complete control of the practice and its operations.

Second Planning Effort between HDI and Medical Groups

Upon reviewing the failure of its initial approach and learning what the groups needed from an affiliation, in May 1991 HDI invited both SJMG and GSMG to hear a new proposal. Less control by HDI, sufficient funds to purchase assets and take over liabilities from each group, expansion funds for group satellites and new office buildings, funds for the recruitment of additional physicians, and significant investment in information systems were included in HDI's new proposal.

The SJMG had already decided to leave the HDI system for another hospital. There had been conflict over HDI's relationship with SJMG in the inpatient risk pool of the managed care contract they had entered jointly. Health Dimensions, Inc., had imposed a fee increase midway through the contract year, eliminating prior savings achieved in the inpatient pool. The SJMG argued that the increases in inpatient reimbursement should not have been instituted until the end of the contract year. Because it was facing significant financial losses, HDI would not change its position. Already SJMG had begun meeting with other hospitals and shifting its patient admissions out of the HDI system.

GSMG, however, accepted the concepts presented. They were committed to developing a partnership with an integrated organization and, based on the new proposal, felt that HDI would be the best partner.

With the signing of a letter of intent, another group of consultants was brought in to educate both the HDI board and the medical group concerning the structure of an integrated system. The consultants emphasized the change required to ensure success under capitated reimbursement, both in the group's practice activities and its utilization of the inpatient facilities. The essential role of the primary care physician in services provided to patients was addressed with both organizations.

Concerted educational efforts were required for HDI and its board to recognize the need to promote outpatient services through the Foundation and accept reduced inpatient utilization. Leaders at HDI also had difficulty letting go of the tradition of serving the entire medical staff without favoring any one group of physicians. At the same time, attorneys were brought in to begin the paperwork for establishing a foundation model and to develop a professional services agreement between the Foundation and the group.

Medical Staff Reaction/Inclusion of IPA

From the beginning of these discussions in 1989, the rest of the medical staff at HDI had been concerned over the development of a foundation, fearing their exclusion from any managed care contracts negotiated by such a foundation. Upon termination of the initial planning effort, the medical staff believed that development of a foundation with the existing groups was a dead issue until they learned of the letter of intent.

Upon learning about the medical staff's negative reaction to the letter of intent, HDI delayed discussions pending investigation to determine whether a foundation structure could be expanded to include a larger segment of the medical staff. The PPO and IPA reviewed the proposal and presented mechanisms for their inclusion in the foundation.

The PPO's presentation reflected its continued resistance to capitated reimbursement, as well as lack of organization or systems for effecting changes in practice patterns or resource utilization. In addition, the majority of PPO membership were specialists and surgeons with little understanding or tolerance of the primary care gatekeeper role. The IPA had demonstrated its ability to control costs in a capitated environment through its experience in the Aetna capitated product, and almost 40 percent of IPA members were primary care physicians. Eventually HDI selected the IPA to participate in the new foundation model; HDI's board hoped this step not only would relieve the medical staff's criticism with regard to forming a foundation but also enhance the geographic distribution of primary care physicians and enable additional patient volume to be managed by the foundation.

Although including the IPA in the foundation allowed planning to move forward, continued objections from the medical staff forced the HDI board to call for the resignations of the hospital system's president and vice-president, both of whom had been CEOs of the system's two original hospitals and had developed the foundation plan. The relationship with the nonfoundation members of the medical staff continues to be an issue for HDI.

In retrospect, this transition of HDI leadership was beneficial in implementing an integrated system. The CEO ultimately selected to lead HDI had previous experience in an integrated model and understood the need for an affiliated group practice to influence change in physician practice patterns in order to succeed in a capitated health care delivery system. He did not have the "baggage" that came with traditional operation of hospitals and quickly focused energies and resources on developing foundation operation as the key element for HDI's survival.

The change in HDI leadership and inclusion of the IPA in the Foundation concerned GSMG, whose members felt that despite the philosophy laid out by HDI, GSMG might not be an equal partner in the Foundation. The GSMG decided to investigate the affiliation efforts SJMG was pursuing with other hospitals. After initial discussions, GSMG decided that SJMG would still demand a dominant role in any joint affiliation and elected to continue discussions with HDI.

☐ Negotiations

Upon GSMG's acceptance of HDI's decision to include the IPA in contracts to provide care to the Foundation's managed care patients, negotiations began for implementation of the Foundation. The GSMG was represented by its physician president, HDI was represented by the senior vice-president, and the IPA was represented by its physician president. Consultants participated in negotiations related to the GSMG and IPA agreement and continued to educate the physicians and HDI leadership. The attorneys negotiated legal issues surrounding development of a foundation model.

Negotiations between physician groups were facilitated by the IPA president and the GSMG president, both of whom shared a strong informal relationship and over the years had discussed physician practices in a changing environment and their respective organizations' approach to dealing with these issues. This personal relationship, which had not existed between GSMG and SJMG, ultimately played a significant role in bringing the two organizations together. In addition, the consultants helped these two organizations recognize that despite differences in their structures (the most significant being the IPA physicians' perception of a loss of autonomy in group practice), both faced similar issues in dealing with capitated reimbursement. Both groups eventually recognized that these issues could be resolved by combining the efforts of these physician organizations with the HDI inpatient system.

Structure

The Foundation was to purchase GSMG assets, operate its practice, and enter into an agreement for GSMG and IPA to provide professional services for the Foundation practice and contracted managed care patients. Also, the Foundation would contract for managed care services for HDI as well as for the medical practices.

As a subsidiary corporation of HDI with its own board of trustees reporting to the HDI board, the Foundation would be at the same organizational level as hospitals in the HDI system and have representation on the HDI board. This way, strategies and resources could be shared, a concept accepted by the group.

Agreement between the GSMG and the IPA

Negotiations between the GSMG and the IPA were difficult and might not have been completed successfully without a consultant. Physicians in the IPA were experiencing varying levels of capitated reimbursement but averaged only 10 to 15 percent prepaid revenues, compared with more than 40 percent in the GSMG. The majority of IPA members sought to maintain autonomy in their practice operations.

The first agreement was that reimbursement to physicians for services rendered to Foundation patients would be the same for GSMG and the IPA practices. Capitation payments for primary care physicians and negotiated fees for specialists and surgeons would be consistent.

Foundation governance and operating committees would have equal representation from GSMG and IPA physicians. Essential to this agreement was consensus that the goal of the Foundation was to develop effective risk sharing, resource utilization, and cost controls to successfully compete for capitated contracts and increase the patient population served by the hospitals and physicians.

Because the Foundation would be responsible for all practice billing for the GSMG, but only the billing for its contracts for the IPA physicians, all reimbursement for professional services would be made to the GSMG. The IPA would contract to provide services to the GSMG, with the Foundation being a cosigner on the agreement with the reserved right to approve any contract changes. As capitated reimbursement grew, IPA physicians could join GSMG, where integrated cost controls and practice pattern changes could be implemented most effectively as the economics of medical practice changed. The GSMG would distribute the income based on services rendered by members of GSMG or the IPA. Internally, GSMG continued to determine individual physician compensation on a salary-based formula for distribution of its share of the reimbursement from the Foundation. The IPA continued to reimburse its member physicians based on the services provided in their individual practices.

Patients were to be assigned to primary care physicians based on patient selection of a physician or geographic preference. Surgical and specialty referrals within GSMG or the IPA were to be determined by the primary care physician. A joint committee would monitor this process and resolve disputes. The structure of this agreement is presented in figure 8-2.

Foundation Governance

The GSMG president also would serve as Foundation president, and the IPA president would chair the Foundation board. The Foundation's board of trustees would consist of the following members:

- Two physician members of the IPA
- Two physician members of the GSMG
- Two representatives of HDI
- One physician from outside the region with experience in managed care contracting and risk sharing
- The CEO (nonphysician) of the Foundation
- One representative of local business

Figure 8-2. Structure of the Managed Care Agreement

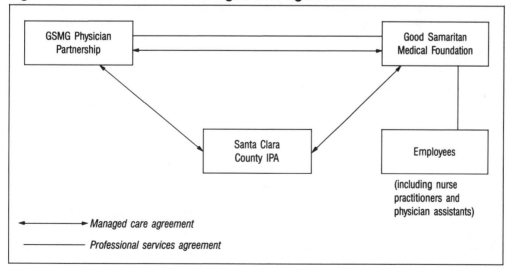

The effort to provide equal representation from the GSMG and the IPA in the leadership was also applied to making committee assignments.

Reimbursement for Physician Services

Initial reimbursement from the Foundation for professional services was set at 50 percent of revenues, based on past and current financial results in the group and on market standards of physician reimbursement by specialty. This reimbursement would be negotiated annually at a rate set on a prospective basis through review of additional factors. Such factors included the number of physicians providing services; the level of care to the medically indigent population; productivity as measured by hours worked, number of enrolled patients, and/or productivity per procedure; and the Foundation's operating costs.

Purchase of the Group Practice

An amount of $15 million was budgeted for purchasing the assets, assuming GSMG liabilities, and funding working capital for Foundation start-up. Hard assets of the GSMG were appraised by an independent consultant, and a fair market value was negotiated. The existing accounts receivable were retained by the group. Contracts and liabilities were transferred to the Foundation.

Financing was obtained through loans from HDI, with a fair market interest rate and payback terms. Tax-exempt financing was not used during initial phases of Foundation formation.

Name of the Foundation

After lengthy negotiation concerning a name for the Foundation, GSMG's insistence that its name recognition be maintained was accepted. The new Foundation, which would be part of the HDI system, was named the Good Samaritan Medical Foundation. The medical group would remain the Good Samaritan Medical Group and contract with the foundation of the same name.

☐ Implementation and Outcomes

The IRS and the California Department of Corporations approved all applications and agreements to form the Good Samaritan Medical Foundation, and the papers were signed on March 31, 1992. Health Dimensions, Inc., was the sole member of the Foundation, with reserved powers given to the Foundation in the corporation documents, including its ability to elect whether to remain with HDI should HDI be sold or merged, as well as its ability to survive and be exempt from any bankruptcy filed by HDI.

In June 1992, a managed care agreement between GSMG and the IPA was approved. This agreement included the description and respective representation on Foundation committees including "manpower," "credentials," "utilization review," and others.

Urgi-Care Centers

Shortly after implementation of the Foundation, the urgi-care centers, which had been managed and staffed by the SJMG, were transferred into the Foundation. These facilities had experienced losses since their start-up as urgi-care centers, and the Foundation quickly approved their transition to primary care centers to become practice sites for the Foundation patients. The Foundation manages the sites, and professional services are provided by GSMG.

Residency Program

As a tax-exempt entity, the Good Samaritan Medical Foundation is required to pursue educational and research activities as part of its operations. A family medicine residency training program, affiliated with the Stanford University School of Medicine (Stanford, CA) and consisting of faculty positions and 18 residency slots, was transferred to the Foundation. This program was expanded to include training sites at facilities in the Foundation practice network.

Management Transition

With turnover of the CEO position at HDI in the fall of 1992, much of the top management personnel at HDI were replaced. A top requirement for replacements was experience in integrated systems. In addition, replacements for management positions have been given dual responsibility within the organizations of the HDI system. Examples of these positions are provided in the following list:

- Chief executive officer of GSMF and vice-president of medical care services for HDI
- Chief financial officer of GSMF and vice-president of finance for HDI
- President of GSMF and president of GSMG
- Chairman of the board for GSMF and president of IPA
- Senior vice-president and chief financial officer of HDI and president of HAV (subsidiary for joint ventures and for-profit activities)
- Senior vice-president for community and home services for HDI and president of subsidiary visiting nurses association

This transition strategy has been important to a smooth integration of operations.

Communications

As part of the implementation, telephone and computer systems were fully integrated among HDI, the Foundation, and GSMG. This was a further step in ensuring ease of communication between the organizations. As a result of this integration, GSMF now performs all managed care contracting for the HDI system. A managed care task force meets regularly with HDI and GSMF executives and physician leaders. In addition, data and outcomes information are easily communicated to and acted upon by committees from both organizations.

Board Composition

Regulations for tax-exempt organizations seeking financing through tax-exempt bond issues required that Board membership *not* exceed 20 percent by physicians involved in the medical services provided by the Foundation. Because initial funding of the Foundation did not include tax-exempt financing, and in order to achieve the goal of committed physician leadership for the Foundation, the nine-member board had four practicing physicians. A ruling on the Friendly Hills Medical Foundation changed the requirements to include this 20 percent limitation on practicing physicians for all tax-exempt medical practice organizations, without the requirement of tax-exempt financing.

In reviewing this new requirement, the Good Samaritan Medical Foundation Board elected to maintain its current physician representation level of four and expand its total membership to 20. New members are selected from the business community *and* from representatives of enrollees in managed care plans that contract with the Foundation for medical services. It is anticipated that this change, dictated by IRS guidelines, will help the Foundation continue to improve its services and marketability to managed care products.

Financial Results

As of September 1993, the Foundation had annual revenues of approximately $30 million, of which 68 percent was from capitated contracts. Six contracts cover 45,000 lives, of which 3,000 are under Medicare risk contracts. The Foundation is aggressively seeking global capitation contracts, where physician services and inpatient care are reimbursed on a prepaid basis, to enhance marketability to capitated plans and develop true risk and reward sharing between the hospital and the physicians.

The Foundation is behind schedule in achieving its goal of breaking even from operations in the third year. The losses in excess of the budget are attributed primarily to the rapid growth of the number of physicians in GSMG and financial losses assumed in incorporating the four HDI urgent care satellite centers in 1992. This issue is being addressed through aggressive growth in capitated patient enrollment, cost reductions through continued integration of resources, capitation of specialists and surgeons, and continued education of physicians on utilization controls.

Physician Growth

The GSMG has grown to 41 physicians and the IPA to 320 members. Despite the fact that one-third of these physicians are in primary care specialties, and despite this being the fastest-growing component of physician membership in both groups, the Foundation leadership is concerned that too many specialists and surgeons are being brought into the practice. It is GSMG's perception that HDI's endorsement of the additional surgeons and specialists is the result of continuing pressure from the rest of the medical staff and those physicians' fears of being excluded from managed care contracts.

Discussions of this issue have led to a decision to provide capitated reimbursement under the Foundation's contracts to surgeons and specialists. Each specialty group has been established into a departmental structure, with leadership represented by physician members from both GSMG and the IPA. The economic impact of capitating these specialists will force each department to control its numbers in the most appropriate way.

GSMG Physician Income Distribution

In 1988 GSMG had developed an income distribution method that provided each physician a base salary and an opportunity to share any group profits based on a productivity formula. The base salary was determined by market compensation rates for each medical and surgical specialty and seniority in the group. The bonus was based on distribution of group profits to individual physicians based on their individual percentage of the group's total productivity.

Shortly after the Foundation was established, GSMG elected to change the bonus incentive of its physician income distribution. A committee of GSMG physicians was established to distribute any profits of the group after physician base salaries were paid according to the following formula:

- 50 percent based on productivity as measured by hours worked, number of primary care patients enrolled, number of patients seen per hour, and relative value of procedures performed by each physician
- 25 percent based on each physician's utilization of resources, weighed by complexity of the patient's problem
- 25 percent based on physician quality as measured by patient survey results, patient wait time, and number of legitimate patient complaints

This change in bonus incentives reflects GSMG's acceptance of the need to change practice patterns as revenues become dominated by capitation.

□ Future Outlook

Despite the management and operational demands of its rapid growth in the first two years, the Foundation has provided leadership for HDI in several areas. These include development of expanded physician services, pursuit of contractual relationships with other provider organizations, and efforts to further integrate health care providers affiliated with HDI. Additional goals include the following:

- *MSO:* The Foundation is developing a management services organization to work with physicians on the HDI medical staff who do not elect to join the IPA or GSMG. Services offered will include billing and information systems, management, staffing, purchasing, operating systems, and so forth. The costs of operating the MSO will be recovered through a management fee to contracted practices. This effort reflects a continued response to the needs of the entire HDI medical staff.
- *Affiliations with other IPAs:* The Good Samaritan Medical Foundation has been approached by other IPA organizations in the San Francisco Bay area to develop affiliations for contracting purposes and for HDI to provide management services. As of this writing, the Foundation manages an IPA outside its service area and has developed an occupational medicine network to provide services to markets immediately surrounding the San Jose/Santa Clara area. Hopefully these efforts will further the Foundation's ability to contract for managed care patients through expanded geographic coverage.
- *Strategic planning:* A joint strategic planning process has been introduced that involves HDI, the Foundation, the GSMG, the IPA, and the remaining HDI subsidiaries (such as a visiting nurse's association). The purpose of this process is to continue to fully integrate all the components of health care delivery under the umbrella of HDI. Part of this planning process includes continued education of the physicians and HDI leaders about the need to change practice patterns and develop new patient management skills. The Good Samaritan Medical Foundation has begun to provide leadership in this planning process. Efforts to implement HDI's strategic goals are growing through the Foundation. By strengthening the Foundation, where governance and financial risk are shared by the hospitals and the physicians, this integrated delivery system looks forward to continued growth and success.

Chapter 9

Millard Fillmore Health System

Shelley Hirshberg, Director of System Development,
Millard Fillmore Health System, Buffalo, NY,
and Daniel Morelli, MD, Vice-Chairman and Clinical Associate
Professor, Department of Family Medicine, and Residency Program
Director, State University of New York at Buffalo, NY

☐ Executive Summary: Key Elements of the Affiliation

- *Organizational structure:* A hospital-owned network of primary care facilities that contracts with a medical school to provide professional services to patients and supervision of teaching and research activities in the group practice network.
- *Hospital goals:* The plan to develop hospital satellite primary care clinics was a result of the Millard Fillmore Health System's goal to enhance its relationship with a medical school by providing primary care training sites and meeting the primary care needs of its service area. Based on success of the initial centers, the hospitals incorporated further development of primary care satellites into their long-range planning. This strategic plan addresses not only continued primary care education and research and service to an underserved population, but also development of an integrated network for the delivery of care under health care reform and changing health care reimbursement through a new affiliated group practice model.
- *Physician needs and goals:* The medical school required additional primary care sites and faculty to expand its education and training of primary care physicians. The hospitals' medical staff were concerned about potential competition from the primary care sites but accepted development of this faculty group practice to meet the teaching needs of the medical school and to serve the indigent population in the service area.
- *Personal relationships:* Strong relationships among the leadership of the medical school, the management, and the family medicine department facilitated the initiation of the primary care satellite clinics, which formed the nucleus for a multisite hospital-affiliated group practice.
- *Health care reform and managed care:* Capitated reimbursement for health care services is anticipated in the Buffalo area. The hospitals' affiliated primary care group has responded to the changing reimbursement environment by actively contracting with various fee-for-service managed care products. State health care reform related to the training of primary care physicians and the meeting of unmet community need for primary services played a major role in the development of this primary care network.

- *Market and competitor activities:* Buffalo is a highly competitive health care environment, and the hospitals are well positioned through their affiliation with the medical school, development of satellite facilities including the primary care network, and affiliations with multiple hospitals. Competitor hospitals have initiated discussion with the Millard Fillmore Health System in part through the success of this primary care network.
- *Capital needs and resources:* The hospitals provided initial funding for development of the primary care practice sites and the recruitment of medical school faculty physicians to staff the sites. The hospitals provide all management services, utilizing existing departments and resources extensively; a division was established to operate the primary care practices.
- *Physician recruitment and retention:* All physicians staffing the primary care network were recruited to the faculty of the medical school. This academic association, as well as competitive compensation packages, has led to successful recruitment and retention of primary care physicians.
- *Legal and contracting issues:* Legal issues were kept to a minimum because the primary care practice sites were developed as extension clinics of the hospital. A contract was developed with the medical school to provide professional staffing in the primary care practices.

☐ Introduction

The Millard Fillmore Gates Circle Hospital was founded in 1872. Located in downtown Buffalo, New York, this 443-bed tertiary care and teaching facility offers a full range of acute care/specialty services and a 75-bed skilled nursing facility. A second hospital, the Millard Fillmore Suburban Hospital, was opened in 1974 and is a 145-bed medical, surgical, and obstetrical hospital located in a growing suburb 15 miles from the Gates Circle facility.

These two hospitals became the Millard Fillmore Health System (the Hospitals), which currently operates 13 freestanding facilities, including three rehabilitation centers; an ambulatory surgery center; a radiology, cardiology, and neurology diagnostic center; a state-of-the-art center for laboratory medicine; five family medicine centers; and two internal medicine primary care centers, in addition to the two original hospitals.

In 1986 the Hospitals established their first primary care center in an office building behind the Millard Fillmore Suburban Hospital. This center was created as part of the Hospitals' strategy to fulfill an educational mission to develop a family medicine residency program in collaboration with the State University of New York at Buffalo's School of Medicine and Bio-Medical Sciences (the University).

By 1993 the five family medicine primary care centers were staffed by 20 family medicine physicians and projected an excess of 40,000 visits annually, generating over 2,500 primary and specialty admissions to the Hospitals. In addition to their educational mission, the primary care centers are considered a very successful component of the mission to "provide quality medical and health care services to meet identified needs of the Western New York community." The fifth center, which opened in November 1993, is not included in this case study.

In addition to achieving the original goal of providing a setting for family medicine postgraduate and medical school training, the primary care centers were a catalyst to change the Hospitals' focus from strictly inpatient-oriented care with traditional outpatient department functions to a primary care focus that addresses the overall needs of the community it serves. Although the centers do not generate a profit from their direct operations, they contribute to hospital activities through direct admissions of patients and referrals to specialists, as well as through use of hospital ancillary services; these revenues offset the hospital investment. In addition, the development of a primary care network and its focus on community needs has positioned the Hospitals as a leader among Western New York health providers as the region begins to experience the impact of health care reform and anticipates managed care contracts and capitated reimbursement.

□ Background

The Hospitals' service area includes Erie and Niagara counties, with a population of 1,164,000. These two counties have experienced a 6 percent decline in population since 1980. Additionally, 15 percent of the population is over age 65, and approximately 24 percent of the total residents are below the poverty level.

In 1986 the Health Systems Agency of Western New York published a plan identifying specific health manpower shortage areas that required primary care services. The study showed that of 253 primary care providers, only 27 full-time-equivalent physicians were dedicated to serve the Medicaid population. The study further reported that physician reluctance to see these patients generally was based on Medicaid reimbursement rates and bureaucratic problems related to obtaining reimbursement for services rendered. This identified community need became central to the planning and implementation of the additional primary care centers by the Millard Fillmore Health System.

Managed care penetration into the market was not a significant factor in the original decision to develop the primary care centers. No capitated contracts were being offered outside a closed-panel HMO introduced in the Buffalo market in 1978. Neither the Hospitals nor their medical staff members participated in this HMO.

Two open-panel HMOs introduced in the market reimburse physicians on a discounted-fee schedule. The Millard Fillmore Health System and its primary care centers provide a substantial portion of care to the more than 400,000 members currently enrolled in these insurance products. State insurance law requires HMOs to enroll Medicaid recipients, and the primary care centers serve as major access points for their enrollment.

Hospital

Historically, the 20 hospitals located in the Buffalo area have been competitive, with minimal collaboration among them. The exception was a consortium of eight hospitals, including the two Millard Fillmore Health System hospitals, created in 1986 that traditionally provided the clinical settings for medical students and graduate medical training programs through the University. The Millard Fillmore Health System considered its affiliation with the medical school a critical factor in maintaining its reputation for high-quality care through teaching and research, as well as its hospitals' ability to maintain a sufficient level of primary and specialty care physicians and services.

The Hospitals' service area includes a significant percentage of patients below the poverty level, most of whom are located near the downtown hospital location. Despite this high percentage of Medicaid patients, through good occupancy levels, the development of tertiary services, and good management, the Hospitals have been financially sound since 1983. The Hospitals are among only 20 hospitals *statewide* with a positive net operating margin.

Medical Staff

The Millard Fillmore Health System's medical staff is dominated by private practitioners in small group or solo practices. Subsequent to the 1986 consortium agreement, several departmental chairmen at the system's hospitals were recruited as joint university–hospital appointments to guide the departmental training of medical students and residents. Other system hospital chairs were filled by voluntary members of the medical staff.

In the mid-1980s, most of the medical staff did not accept indigent patients in their private practices. Instead they served in hospital-based teaching clinics, providing care to this population segment as part of their voluntary faculty obligation to teach medical students and postgraduate students.

Traditionally the medical staff supported the Hospitals' involvement in medical education and resident training and unanimously supported enhancement of these activities. Creation of the consortium, however, did cause some concern among the medical staff that the University and its faculty might eventually dominate the Hospitals' medical staff affairs. These fears were offset by the credibility the consortium brought to the institution and its medical staff and by the limited, noncompetitive role of full-time University faculty.

☐ Motivations for Primary Care Center Development

Three key motivators spurred development of primary care centers. They were the opportunities to introduce family medicine education to the Hospitals; serve the indigent population; and develop a core of loyal primary care physicians.

Introducing Family Medicine Postgraduate Education

To achieve the goal of introducing family medicine postgraduate education, consensus was required between the University's school of medicine and the Hospitals' board and medical staff. In developing the first primary care center, the University wanted to expand its family medicine postgraduate training into the Hospitals, needed to fund development and expansion of its faculty base, and desired to become less dependent on a single hospital setting in which to provide its family medicine resident training. University funds to support faculty salaries, benefits, and development were limited. Reimbursement for patient services rendered by the faculty at the primary care center could serve as a source of these needed funds.

Serving Indigent Populations

Millard Fillmore Health System was motivated to develop a primary care network to achieve its mission of meeting the needs of its underserved populations. This could be achieved through the activities of a family medicine training program. Moreover, an affiliation with the University could bring financial support to the effort through income generated by residents in the outpatient and inpatient settings, grants, reimbursement for training costs, and research funding.

Developing a Core of Loyal Primary Care Providers

The Hospitals also saw the primary care centers as vehicles for developing a solid core of primary care providers whose loyalty to the Millard Fillmore Health System would be ensured by virtue of their joining the Hospitals' medical staff upon graduation from the program. The medical staff believed that the family medicine training program would provide primary care to the indigent patient group, allowing the private practitioners on staff to focus on insured, paying patients in their practices. In addition, referrals to specialists at the Hospitals would be enhanced through the increased number of patients seen at the new training site. The medical staff was concerned about University presence in the Hospitals and potential competition for patients in the community. These concerns were counterbalanced by the previously noted financial benefits to the medical staff, the quality of faculty who staffed the centers, and the noncompetitive services that the faculty would provide to the underserved populations.

☐ Planning for Initial Primary Care Center

Planning for the first primary care center began in 1983. Key players in this process were the CEO of the Millard Fillmore Health System, the chairman of the University's department of family medicine, and the former chairman of the department of family medicine at the Hospitals. The latter had long championed the development of a family medicine postgraduate program for the Hospitals during his private practice activities and membership on the medical staff. The respect with which he was held among the Hospitals' medical staff members was essential in maintaining their commitment to initiate this program.

It was understood from the start that the Hospitals would provide the financial support needed for the capital, operating, and faculty costs for the training program. The University had no funds for development and staffing of a primary care center that could provide an ambulatory care experience in a consistent setting over a three-year training period for its residents.

Physicians

Direct employment of physicians by the Hospitals was rejected because the University needed to develop and direct the teaching program. In addition, there was concern over possible medical staff objections to the Hospitals' employment of physicians in a practice that potentially would compete with them. It was finally determined that the physicians who would staff the center should be faculty members, hired by the University's department of family medicine faculty practice plan. The Hospitals would support the salary and benefits of this faculty through a contract with the practice plan.

Ownership and Operations

The center was to be owned and operated by the Hospitals as an extension clinic, a structure that would facilitate the center's start-up funding and operations. Furthermore, based on research findings, total Medicaid patient reimbursement for primary care services would be greater in a hospital clinic than in a private practice office. The Hospitals would bill for all outpatient and inpatient services provided by the center's medical staff, and the revenue from these services would offset the center's operating expenses, including physicians' salaries and benefits.

A certificate-of-need (CON) application was submitted for approval to develop an extension clinic of the Hospitals. In New York, key criteria for CON approval included the projected level of indigent services, a quantifiable objective that easily could be met under the projections for the center. The University and the Hospitals began the application process for approval as a residency training program.

Business Plan

The measures for success of the first center were not financially oriented; rather, they stressed the importance of education and provision of care to the community. This focus represented a shift from the traditional focus of introducing new services based on inpatient revenues to a recognition of the Hospitals' obligation to provide primary care to its *total* population. Financial projections for the new center did include the elements of additional business that would be brought to the Hospitals and their ancillary departments. Since their inception, this recognition of the primary care centers' financial impact on the entire Millard Fillmore Health System has been a key consideration in reviewing their financial results. A summary of the financial analysis applied to the centers is shown in table 9-1.

Table 9-1. Financial Analysis of Primary Care Centers

	1987	1988	1989	1990	1991	1992	1993
Number of centers	1	1	2	4	4	4	4
Revenue							
Gross outpatient revenue	$16,750	$248,715	$741,017	$1,308,405	$1,255,497	$1,469,680	$2,360,476
Contractual allowance	(1,173)	(17,410)	(37,095)	(26,467)	9,855	29,505	129,180
Net outpatient revenue	15,577	231,305	703,922	1,281,938	1,265,352	1,499,185	2,489,656
Net margin from inpatient admissions	2,847	70,080	183,084	319,521	327,624	356,751	580,788
Total net revenue	18,424	301,385	887,006	1,601,459	1,592,976	1,855,936	3,070,444
Expenses							
Salaries	137,612	231,910	428,846	623,203	699,512	804,324	1,165,691
Fringes	18,578	31,308	59,181	97,220	109,124	125,475	181,848
Professional fees	31,161	84,991	275,242	378,336	471,941	601,521	1,203,713
Supplies	7,870	12,387	25,599	50,925	45,517	82,784	116,424
Other expense	98,166	89,990	159,037	245,741	286,017	318,052	442,526
Total expense	293,387	450,586	947,905	1,395,425	1,612,111	1,932,156	3,110,202
Net gain (loss)	(274,963)	(149,201)	(60,899)	206,034	(19,135)	(76,220)	(39,758)
Capital investment	(279,462)	0	(149,085)	(282,363)	(8,225)	(95,000)	0
Return on investment	(554,425)	(149,201)	(209,984)	(75,329)	(27,360)	(171,220)	(39,758)
Cumulative return on investment	(554,425)	(703,626)	(913,610)	(988,939)	(1,016,299)	(1,187,519)	(1,227,277)

□ Negotiations

With the agreement that the Hospitals would receive the revenues from the primary care centers and be responsible for the majority of funding, negotiations with the medical school began in earnest. Issues addressed included physician compensation and support related to both academic and practice requirements, management, and location of the first practice site.

Physician Compensation

A major element of the negotiations was the compensation paid to the faculty practice plan for the teaching and patient care activities of faculty physicians. Again, it was understood that revenues from patient services provided at the center and in the Hospitals would have to finance this program.

Upon analysis of the components of teaching and patient care, it was determined that a full-time physician should have 10 half-day work sessions each week. Seven of these sessions would be devoted to patient services, and three would be used to precept, lecture, and counsel medical students and residents and to complete administrative tasks.

In 1986 annual salaries for full-time family medicine faculty were established between $65,000 and $70,000 based on comparative research of starting salaries of Western New York family medicine physicians and faculty positions at other medical schools. By 1990 starting salaries were $90,000 to $95,000 for graduating residents, reflecting the market demand for primary care physicians. An additional $5,000 was paid to faculty physicians providing obstetrical care. Faculty physicians were expected to work 45 weeks per year, with five weeks of vacation and holiday time and two weeks of continuing medical education time.

The Hospitals fund 100 percent of compensation and a percentage of administrative overhead expenses of the University's department of family medicine. In addition, the Hospitals support all costs for recruitment and relocation of new faculty members. The department uses funds from research grants and the University to cover additional overhead expenses and to offset some faculty salaries.

Negotiations also led to a patient volume–based incentive program for staff physicians, which was not implemented until the center's third year due to the uncertainty of patient activity projections during the planning and start-up process. The incentive program provided for a percentage of net revenues generated from patient volume that exceeded target volume to be included in the payment to the faculty practice plan. After two years, this program was discontinued due to the faculty's negative perceptions of productivity levels used as a standard in a teaching environment. The Hospitals and the University department are developing quality and productivity standards effective for 1994 application to the clinical components of the faculty's obligations at the centers.

Management

Because of the initial emphasis on development and implementation of the teaching program in conjunction with the primary care centers' patient services, overall responsibility for implementation and operation of the center fell to the University's department of family medicine. A vice-chairman was hired and appointed chairman of family medicine at the Hospitals and made medical director of the first primary care center. His compensation was funded jointly by the Hospitals and the University.

Site Selection

A medical office building adjacent to the Millard Fillmore Suburban Hospital was selected because of the space availability and access to the hospital. Increased enrollment of the population surrounding the hospital in managed care plans in which the faculty would participate was also considered. With approval of the CON and the residency program, renovations began in 1986.

☐ Implementation

Neither the Hospitals nor the University had built or operated a freestanding primary care center and no guidelines existed for operating such a facility. Because education was a key priority, the Hospitals gave the medical director a great deal of autonomy in implementing operations. However, the demands for a curriculum, preceptors, and specialty rotations related to establishing a postgraduate training program consumed the majority of his time and energy. The Hospitals' personnel staffing the center were expected to develop operating policies and procedures under the guidance of the center's medical director.

Hospital policies, financial reporting, and billing systems already in place were inpatient oriented. Systems were neither user-friendly nor geared for small physician group practices, and policies were directed toward the more steady work flow and routine of inpatient services. Outpatient billing procedures also needed to be developed.

Initially, the extra work required to meet the demands of what appeared to be a private physician office were not well received by the Hospitals' personnel. The development of such basic services as housekeeping, mail service, purchasing, personnel services, and billing were hindered by this resistance. Only after several years of experience and expansion of the centers did the Hospitals' personnel accept that these centers were truly an extension of the Hospitals. Even today, with seven centers in operation (including the internal medicine centers and a fifth family health center opened in November 1993), many support services are not routinely provided by the Hospitals' support departments but are negotiated with outside vendors.

The supervisor of the primary care center devoted much energy to addressing these issues of incorporating the practice support activities into hospital department functions. Support from the medical director and the administration of the Hospitals was essential in gaining department support for the first center's operating systems.

☐ Outcomes

After the second primary care center opened in 1988, planning for the ongoing development of the centers was incorporated into the strategic planning process for the Hospitals. The success of the postgraduate training programs (the first group of residents completed training in 1989), as well as the volume of patients being treated at the centers, had made them an important part of the Hospitals' operations. The primary motivation for additional centers had shifted to meeting community need, and additional site selection was based on the criteria of identified need for primary care services and minimal competition with the existing medical staff rather than the needs of the teaching programs. In determining the locations for the primary care centers, access to public transportation lines and adequate parking were important considerations.

Planning for Additional Centers

An integral component of the Hospitals' strategic planning process was the development of a database and an environmental assessment. Inpatient statistics, outpatient activities, health status indicators, and service area demographics were analyzed each year as part of the strategic plan. Input from regional health care planning agencies was an integral component of the environmental analysis.

The Hospitals' strategic plans from 1990 through 1993 reflected a specific goal of providing primary care to the underserved, indigent population through development of several additional primary care centers. These additional centers also enabled the University and Hospitals to expand teaching opportunities for medical, nursing, social work, and nutrition students involved in the care delivery at the primary care centers.

The positive results demonstrated by the centers in providing access to care for a previously underserved population, as well as their participation in managed care products, made the centers a leading resource for patient services to the Hospitals' service area population. This success is reflected in the payer mix detailed in table 9-2. The 1990 strategic plan includes a section titled "Access to Care" that incorporates the activities of the primary care centers. (See figure 9-1.)

The number of physicians in each zip code area was studied to determine the areas of need for center sites. The Health System Agency's primary needs analysis, which was

Table 9-2. Primary Care Centers Payer Mix

	1990/1991	1993
Medicaid	34.5%	44.5%
Medicaid managed care	N/A	7.9%
Medicare	14.1%	14.9%
Self-pay	5.2%	4.4%
Non-Medicaid managed care	N/A	18.4%
Commercial	46.2%	9.9%

broader than the physician analysis in looking at medically underserved areas (state and federally designated), was incorporated. Physicians in each zip code were also studied to determine who among them accepted Medicaid patients in general and, specifically, which physicians were accepting new Medicaid patients. Initial planning efforts involved the Hospitals' *primary service area* only, which was defined as the pool from which 80 percent of inpatient admissions were generated. Currently, the Hospital is looking outside its immediate service area to other areas with indigent underserved populations.

Nonphysician Staffing

Initially, nonphysician staffing of the centers reflected the Hospitals' lack of experience in managing a freestanding medical practice operation. Due to the ambiguity in New York State health codes related to hospital extension clinics, every center is staffed with a full-time registered nurse and full-time clinical and clerical support. As patient volume increased at the centers, support staff were added incrementally. Some differences in staffing occurred based on the community served and activities at each of the sites. For example, residency training sites have additional secretarial support for the training program; the center that serves the Hispanic community employs several translators to assist

Figure 9-1. Excerpt from Millard Fillmore Hospitals' 1990 Strategic Plan

---

Issue III. Access to Care

Corporate Goal 1.

Millard Fillmore Hospitals will continue to provide health care services to medically underserved neighborhoods and enhance the continuity of patient care through a variety of support services.

Strategy Statements

1. Establish primary care extension clinics in underserved neighborhoods.
2. Assist primary care physicians to develop practices in underserved areas.
3. Recruit physicians from the University Family Medicine Residency program and Millard Fillmore Hospitals' Medicine Residency program.
4. Work with Information Services to facilitate data gathering for planning, clinical, and research purposes.
5. Expand existing [support services] and develop new support services as appropriate for patient care activities in the outpatient areas.
6. Develop collaborative efforts with other health care providers and community agencies as appropriate to enhance access to care.

Corporate Goal 2.

Enhance awareness of Millard Fillmore Hospitals' philosophy on care to indigent and access issues to create mechanisms to deal with improving access.

Strategy Statements

1. Network with businesses and members of the neighborhood community.
2. Formalize an "Access to Care" committee process by activating, on an ongoing basis, specific Task Force groups to address issues such as transportation, language, facility, and financial barriers.
3. Respond in a timely fashion to all appropriate financial initiatives put forth by the New York State Department of Health and by any federally mandated programs.
4. Define programs that will educate Millard Fillmore Hospitals' employees regarding issues of access and the cultural needs of our patients.

Corporate Goal 3.

Millard Fillmore Hospitals will support the long-range primary care plans of the Departments of Medicine and Family Medicine.

Strategy Statements

1. Restructure outpatient services to ensure that the immediate community's needs are met in addition to the training needs of all primary care residency programs.
2. Evaluate on a regular basis all primary care programs to ensure success in meeting targeted utilization levels.

---

non-Spanish-speaking staff, as well as a phlebotomist due to the high volume of laboratory work done at this site.

Staffing strategy addresses the need to increase operating efficiencies at the centers. A proposal is under consideration to allocate staff based on standards for a private physician's office practice. This staffing pattern would provide two staff members, clinical and clerical, for every full-time-equivalent physician to support patient care activities. The goal is to train all nonlicensed staff as medical office assistants to assume support functions to meet the business and clinical needs of the faculty physicians and allow for cross-coverage of staffing across all centers.

Registered nurses at each center would focus on patient education and patient compliance with treatment plans for all of the center's patients, a major issue in providing care to indigent populations. The unique needs of each center continue to be met with additional staff at the site, shared by all of the physicians' practices.

Center Management

The administrative structure of center operations has evolved since the first center opened. As more centers were developed it became clear that the Hospitals needed a centralized management structure for operations. By 1990 four centers had opened. Medical directors were designated for each site, and the chairperson of the Hospitals' family medicine department was given responsibility for coordination of their activities. A new position, assistant administrator for outreach and ambulatory care services, was created and filled by an individual from the center's administrative office. Figure 9-2 shows the current

Figure 9-2. Organizational Chart, Primary Care Centers

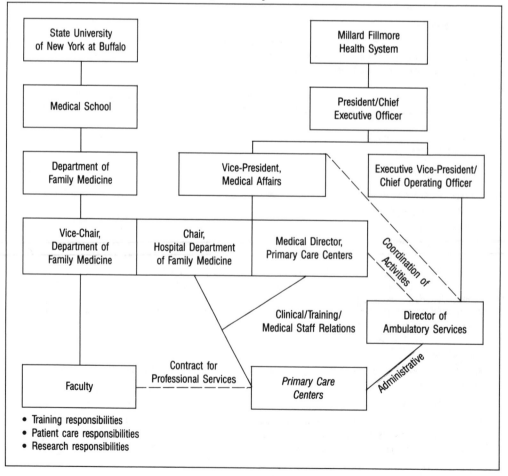

- Training responsibilities
- Patient care responsibilities
- Research responsibilities

organizational structure. In 1991 two new administrative positions were created: an administrative director and director of nursing for all primary care center operations.

In November 1993, a coordinator position was created for each center and charged with supervision of day-to-day operations and collaboration with that center's medical directors. Depending on the center's volume and operational needs, the goal is for the clinic coordinators to spend 70 percent of time participating in business and/or clinical functions and 30 percent providing management support. As mentioned previously, the current focus is to maximize office efficiencies and productivity.

Patient Volume

Most of the centers were built to accommodate four full-time physicians. The full-time faculty physicians spend approximately seven sessions lasting three and one-half hours each providing outpatient care in the centers, two sessions teaching courses and/or precepting the residents, and one session fulfilling administrative tasks. It is expected that a primary care physician with this profile would see approximately 3,700 patients per year. Therefore, it is projected that each center will accommodate at least 15,000 to 18,000 visits per year. The volume of patient visits for the four primary care centers is reflected in figure 9-3.

Physician Recruitment and Employment

As centers were added, expertise grew in terms of planning and setting up facilities and operations, with the self-limiting factor being in the area of physician recruitment, which warranted a full-time physician recruiter. Since this position was created in November 1991, 13 family medicine physicians have been recruited to staff the centers. Three reasons account for this successful recruitment effort. The first was the focused effort of the recruiter on primary care recruitment; the second was the desirability of the academic model; and the third was the community-oriented approach in the centers' mission.

Medical Staff Acceptance

As development of the centers has progressed, the medical staff has accepted that the centers do not compete for private practice patients, and the growth in patient volumes has demonstrated the need for additional primary care providers in the area. Figure 9-4 is a graph of inpatient admissions generated by the centers. As anticipated by the original planners, many medical staff members acknowledge that their practices have been

Figure 9-3. Primary Care Centers Outpatient Visits

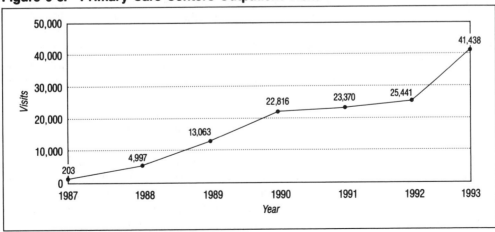

Figure 9-4. Inpatient Admissions Generated by Primary Care Centers

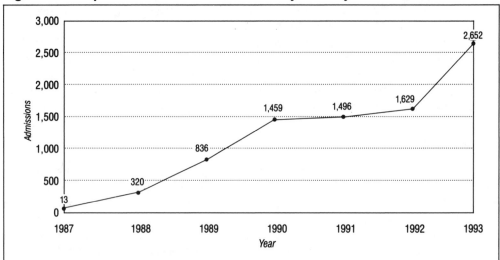

Note: Admissions are generated directly by primary care physicians and specialty referrals from the primary care centers.

enhanced by center referrals, further serving to eliminate the earlier concern over the Hospitals' employment of physicians at the centers. Development of two internal medicine centers by the Hospitals did include Hospital-employed physicians, without objection from the medical staff.

Continued Planning

Every two years an image survey is conducted by the Millard Fillmore Health System. Also, a detailed health assessment of the communities for the purpose of identifying the true health care needs and desires is planned. The image surveys have concluded that the patient population considers OB/GYN as primary care (obstetrics is part of the family medicine training) and that there remains a need to provide culturally sensitive, accessible primary care services. The employment of staff (including physicians) with ethnic, cultural, and language backgrounds similar to the population served by the center is a priority.

Relationship with Other Hospitals

After the opening of a primary care center in the North Tonawanda community in the spring of 1990, the local community hospital became concerned about losing patients to Millard Fillmore Hospitals. The community hospital was meeting with difficulty in recruiting and retaining physicians in its community, which was also considered part of the Millard Fillmore Health System's service area. The opening of this center brought the two hospitals to the negotiation table, with the result being that the community hospital realized that the Hospitals had developed a model that enabled them not only to recruit primary care physicians, but also to retain them in the centers. Discussions between the two hospitals have addressed the possibility of merger and/or affiliation. In January 1993, the Millard Fillmore Health System's primary care center was relocated into a 5,000-square-foot space in that community hospital.

Similar collaborations are being discussed with a hospital on the west side of Buffalo, where the Niagara Family Health Center opened in 1988. Until recently, this hospital had not acknowledged the Hospitals' ability to meet the needs of the Hispanic community on the west side of Buffalo. It took five years to overcome resistance to exploring collaborative programs that potentially benefit the Hispanic community.

☐ Future Outlook

Although the Millard Fillmore Health System's primary care initiative was not driven by a cooperative model, it helped to initiate cooperative efforts with other hospitals. Future goals for the primary care centers include the following:

- Continued improvement of productivity, profitability, and performance at all centers through management operations improvements and resource utilization
- Development of an outcomes-oriented database in order to continue adapting patient care delivery to a capitated reimbursement environment
- Continued enhancement of benefits to the University department of family medicine, including provision of:
  - A stable source of funding for faculty expansion
  - Teaching sites for residents and medical students
  - Successful joint recruitment of faculty
  - An effective departmental administrative structure
  - Faculty and clinic site development in primary care teaching and research
- Expansion of ancillary and outreach programs in the centers, including social work, nutrition counseling, and nursing
- Development of an integrated network of primary care physicians for managed care contracting
- Continued development of efficient, high-quality medical care models for the medically underserved and indigent communities

Chapter 10

The Mercy Hospital of Pittsburgh

Irene McFadden, Vice-President, Ambulatory and General Services, Mercy Hospital, Pittsburgh, PA

☐ Executive Summary: Key Elements of the Affiliation

- *Organizational structure:* A hospital-owned and operated group practice works in satellite facilities with hospital-employed physicians.
- *Hospital goals:* The hospital had a need to develop satellite primary care facilities in order to provide access for patients under a hospital-owned HMO product. In addition, this tertiary care hospital and teaching center had identified a strategic need to expand its primary care base to ensure continued referrals to its specialty services.
- *Physician needs and goals:* Most of the medical staff of The Mercy Hospital endorsed expansion of the primary care base as referral sources to their practices. The internal medicine department objected strongly to the development of the family medicine department.
- *Personal relationships:* The hospital experienced difficulty in recruiting a strong chairman for its new family medicine department. This was due in part to the previously mentioned resistance from the internal medicine department.
- *Health care reform and managed care:* The anticipated growth of capitated reimbursement in the Pittsburgh market had led the hospital to develop a partnership with an HMO product. Although this product did not succeed, the primary care group has been a strong vehicle in the hospital's contracting with managed care products.
- *Capital needs and resources:* Because the primary sites were operated as hospital clinics, their capital and start-up funding was provided by the hospital.
- *Physician recruitment and retention:* Recruiting new physicians to the primary care sites initially was difficult because the family medicine department was new and did not have strong leadership. This, coupled with a change in physician compensation from an incentive arrangement to a straight salary, led to physician turnover.
- *Legal and contracting issues:* Legal issues were kept to a minimum because the primary care sites were established as hospital clinics and the physicians were employed.

□ Introduction

The Mercy Hospital of Pittsburgh is a 524-bed, advanced teaching and referral Catholic facility founded in 1847. Located in downtown Pittsburgh, Mercy offers a full range of general medical and surgical services, with specialty programs in cardiac care, cancer care, trauma and burn, and women's and children's services.

During a strategic planning effort conducted in the early 1980s, Mercy recognized that a large percentage of admissions to the hospital were made by specialist members of the medical staff. These specialists depended on referrals from private primary care physicians located in the suburbs, primarily south of Pittsburgh. Many of these physicians were not members of Mercy's medical staff and had no formal association with the hospital. Managed care, in the form of HMOs, had begun to enroll higher percentages of the local population. Mercy historically had a large internal medicine department but no family practice physicians.

Mercy announced the initiation of a department of family practice in 1984, coupled with a decision to develop a network of family health centers in suburban locations. Both actions were taken to allow Mercy's participation in HMO development. The first center, staffed by family practice physicians, was opened in fall 1986; the second facility followed in January 1988. By 1993 the two centers were staffed by 10 family practice physicians and accounted for approximately 14,500 visits each, as well as more than 100 admissions to the hospital.

Since 1993 the Mercy family centers have been considered by the hospital to be a successful enterprise. Although the direct revenues from center operations continue to fall short of direct operating expenses, the overall financial contribution of the centers to the hospital is considered positive in that they generate a steady stream of referrals to hospital-based specialists and ancillary departments. In addition to providing accessible, convenient health care in local communities not historically served by the hospital, the centers ensure a primary care base necessary for appropriate patient care management. Further, the centers enable a range of hospital ancillary and specialty services to be provided in the local community as an adjunct to the family practice sites.

□ Background

Pittsburgh rests in the center of Allegheny County. Between 25 and 30 independent hospitals operated in the county during the early 1980s. Seven of these were considered to be teaching, referral facilities. Traditionally, the hospitals within Allegheny County viewed the geographic area contiguous to their facility as their "owned" service area. The numerous community hospitals, through medical staff referral relationships, had aligned themselves almost exclusively with one or another of the urban teaching facilities.

Pittsburgh had a long history of community health planning (as opposed to competition), and it was common for hospitals to discuss their plans openly and to respect each other's service areas and established lines of referral. However, the local Health Systems Agency had determined that Allegheny County was "over-bedded," population growth was stagnant, and competition for patients was increasing. For example, there had been some experimentation with urgent care centers in Pittsburgh, and Mercy had experienced one failed effort in this area.

By the early 1980s, managed care had made little impact in the Pittsburgh health care marketplace. Less than 12 percent of residents were enrolled in HMOs. However, rapid expansion of the HMO concept was anticipated, and Mercy Hospital had determined that it would develop its own HMO product.

Physicians, including Mercy's medical staff, practiced largely in small, single-specialty groups, or as solo practitioners. A majority of Mercy's attending physicians had their primary office located on the hospital campus. Physicians who had an additional site tended to set up practice in the suburbs south of the city.

Hospital

During the early 1980s, hospital operating margins were solid (approaching 10 percent), but an erosion of margin was anticipated as DRG rates were tightened and managed care expanded. Mercy worked with its medical staff to establish a MeSH (medical staff/hospital) organization, a concept introduced by Paul Ellwood of Intergroup (Minneapolis) and designed to enable joint venturing between a hospital and its staff. The leadership of Mercy's MeSH—later named Mercy Health United—decided to develop a jointly owned HMO in anticipation of expanding the concept in the Pittsburgh market.

Both the MeSH and the HMO were actively supported by the hospital's administration, as well as by the president of the medical staff (an influential member of the private surgical staff) and the chairman of the department of medicine (who became the first medical director of the HMO). Collaboration within the medical staff and between the administration and the medical staff was generally positive and active at the time.

Medical Staff

Mercy Hospital subspecialists, particularly in the surgical specialties, were strong supporters of the HMO concept. They were concerned about ensuring a flow of patients from primary care into their specialty practices. Although the majority of Mercy's medical staff practices continued to experience a steady stream of referrals, they were concerned about potential redirection of that flow as managed care evolved.

The Mercy HMO, later called The HMO Alliance, was regarded as one strategy for ensuring patient flow. However, the medical staff, with the exception of internal medicine, also identified the need to expand the number of primary care practitioners associated with Mercy. Toward this end, in 1984 the medical executive committee recommended that a department of family practice be initiated at Mercy. The recommendation was approved, with a minority objection by the department of internal medicine. The vote was supported by the hospital board of trustees, and the first chair of the department of family practice was recruited in 1985.

☐ Planning

Planning for the family health centers evolved out of the HMO development discussions. The hospital's strategic plan, adopted in 1985, called for the development of ambulatory health care centers in selected geographic locations. The objectives of this initiative included:

- Establishment of a primary care referral base to be formally linked to Mercy's specialty and subspecialty services
- Geographic distribution of Mercy-controlled health care services, providing better access to the Mercy system
- Elimination of geographic gaps in the HMO alliance delivery and primary care service network, thereby improving the overall marketability of the HMO
- Creation of an environment that fosters the evolution of a multispecialty group practice at Mercy

These objectives served as a guide in determining the location, structure, and staffing of the initial family health centers.

Center Locations

Mercy's existing medical staff offices were well distributed throughout the suburbs south of Pittsburgh but were poorly represented in the North Hills area as well as east of the city. Both areas are densely populated by employees of businesses and corporations located in downtown Pittsburgh, to whom the HMO would be marketed. Community hospitals to the east and north of Pittsburgh were contacted to discuss participation in the HMO's development, but none were interested. Mercy decided to proceed independently with the establishment of centers; the first one to be developed in the east, with one to the north to follow within one year.

Market research was conducted to determine specific location and service mix for each center. Data were gathered for each of the target sectors of Allegheny County, including competitor information, a broad range of demographic data, physician-to-population ratios, as well as traffic volumes and availability of appropriate real estate or rental space. The data were organized by township and compared with predetermined criteria designed to help select the specific target site.

Criteria for selecting target locations included:

- Absence of existing Mercy primary care physicians (particularly internists) within specific area to be served
- Ratio of population to primary care physician greater than 20,000 to 1
- Average household income greater than $20,000
- Average house value greater than $60,000
- Less than 7.5 percent of the population over age 65
- Traffic volume on major artery greater than 25,000 cars per day
- Significant total population density within 20 minutes' driving time
- Nearest urgent care center or emergency room farther than four miles away

Additional research of households in the targeted areas was conducted by telephone survey of 400 residents of each targeted area. Research objectives focused on determining insurance coverage, type of physician most frequently used, how the household chooses a physician, satisfaction with current physician care and service, preferred days and hours of physician service availability, ratings of various nearby hospitals (including Mercy), and willingness to change providers if certain practice criteria are met.

The market research supported the conclusion that specific areas east and north of Pittsburgh could benefit from the opening of health care centers that met certain criteria. Specifically, the centers should emphasize service by offering extended evening and weekend hours and care for the entire family (family practice). An additional criterion was that the centers should be identified with Mercy Hospital given that the hospital enjoyed a positive reputation in both areas, although residents to the north viewed Mercy as possibly being too far geographically to go to for admission.

Center Structure

An outside firm was engaged to assist with the financial analysis and the legal issues associated with the centers. Three primary structure alternatives were considered: (1) for-profit subsidiaries of the Pittsburgh Mercy Health System; (2) not-for-profit subsidiaries of Mercy Hospital; and (3) cost centers of Mercy Hospital.

At the time, hospitals continued to receive reimbursement from Medicare and Blue Cross on a cost basis for outpatient services. The hospital cost center approach was determined to be the appropriate short-term structure to ensure maximum reimbursement for the projected payer mix. This would be reexamined if the mix changed or if payment methodologies were altered.

Despite the HMO strategy, in the initial years the majority of patients projected to be seen at the centers fell into two payer categories—Medicare and Blue Cross. Initial payer mix assumptions and actual performance are shown in table 10-1. It was further assumed that as Mercy's HMO became established and achieved its marketing objectives, it would account for an increasing percentage of the centers' activity.

Table 10-1. Family Health Centers Payer Mix

Payer	Assumption (%)	1992 Performance (%)
Medicare	15	10.5
Medicaid	20	11.5
Blue Cross	35	37.0
Commercial	15	15.0
Workers' compensation	8	4.5
Managed care	2	3.0
Self-pay	15	18.5

Physician Staffing

The approach to staffing the ambulatory health centers became the most political issue associated with their development. Members of Mercy's department of internal medicine saw the centers as an opportunity to provide practice sites for residents newly graduated from that department's residency program. However, market research showed that consumers preferred a center with services for patients of all ages, including pediatric patients. The cost of staffing the centers with internists and pediatricians was prohibitive, whereas family practice physicians provided a cost-effective approach to meeting consumer requirements. Despite the department of medicine's lack of support, plans were made to proceed with two family practice sites, a key condition of site selection being that no center be located where Mercy internal medicine practices existed within the target community.

Based on research of typical family practice offices, initial assumptions showed the centers could achieve an average of 50 visits per day within the first year, with 1.8 percent of visits resulting in hospital admissions on a yearly basis. Both surgical and medical subspecialists, recognizing the potential positive impact of this new stream of patients on their practices, supported the family health center concept throughout the process.

Plan Approval

On May 15, 1986, the hospital board of trustees approved the detailed plan to establish the Mercy Family Health Centers, beginning in the eastern suburbs. Specifics of the plan included the following:

- The program would be established as a cost center of the hospital rather than as an independent entity.
- The facility would be leased rather than owned; this decision would be reevaluated after the initial five years of operation.
- The center would be staffed by three full-time family practice physicians, to be salaried and employed by the hospital.
- The center would be designed to include adequate space for the family practice and basic laboratory and radiology services; a conference/meeting area; a procedure room; and additional office and examination space that would be available for rental by specialists.
- The center would be identified as an extension of Mercy Hospital and direct mail used to inform the community about the center and its program offerings.
- Support staff in the center would be hospital employees whose wages and benefits would be consistent with the hospital program.
- Center hours of operation would emphasize convenience and accessibility. Therefore, initially the centers were to be open seven days and six evenings per week.

☐ Implementation

Several issues were addressed as implementation got under way. These included physical space, challenges of physician recruitment and retention, establishment of strong leadership, physician compensation and incentive packages, development of specialty and support services, and HMO participation. How each of these issues was addressed is covered in the following sections.

Facility Design and Capital Equipment

A lease for the first Mercy Family Health Center (the East Center) was negotiated for approximately 7,000 square feet of retail space in a building that is part of a complex located on the major commercial artery in the eastern suburbs. A bidding process led to selection of the architect and contractor for building improvements.

Capital equipment and furnishing needs were determined in consultation with the architect. Most aspects of this phase of implementation proceeded as planned and within budget.

The second center, in the northern suburbs (the North Center), was planned for a fall 1987 opening. Its design was adjusted to resolve specific design issues identified after the east facility opened—for example, inclusion of an additional nursing station to accommodate specialty practice activity. Otherwise, the North Center was planned and initiated within the same general parameters as the East Center. Figure 10-1 summarizes the capital development costs of these first two centers.

The most significant difference in the opening of the second facility was that the building was to be newly constructed, with the Mercy Family Health Center to be the anchor tenant on the first floor. Due to the new construction and weather-related delays, the North Center opened a few months later than scheduled, January 1988.

Physician Recruitment and Retention

The biggest challenge in establishing the first Mercy Family Health Center was recruitment of the medical staff. The chairman of the family practice department had been recruited from outside the Pittsburgh area and had no established relationships with local family practice residency programs. Therefore a recruitment firm was engaged to help identify and select appropriate staff physicians.

There was some difficulty in attracting candidates because of Mercy's limited history with family practice. In addition, members of the department of medicine continued to withhold support for the development of family practice. Potential candidates, concerned over how new the venture was, also sensed the disapproval on the part of medical

Figure 10-1. Capital Development Costs for Family Health Centers

East Center, December 1986	
Facility improvements	$270,000
Equipment and furnishings	177,000
Other preopening expense[a]	119,600
Total	$566,600
North Center, January 1988	
Facility improvements	$322,000
Equipment and furnishings	210,000
Other preopening expense[a]	148,000
Total	$680,000

[a]Advertising, legal and accounting services, recruitment, training, and salaries for support staff and physicians.

staff. By the time construction was complete and the first center was ready to open (November 1986), only two of the three medical staff positions were filled. Interim physicians were engaged to complete the staffing until a full physician complement could be retained.

Despite the atmosphere of transience and lack of continuity in department leadership (described in the next section), volume within the centers grew steadily each month. Physician recruitment continued in efforts to fill three positions for the opening of the second center. By the time the second center was opened, six full-time family practice physicians had been retained.

Unfortunately, once all the staff positions had been filled, the centers began to experience physician turnover. A physician stayed an average of 18 months to two years and then left for another position. Analysis of turnover trends revealed the following profile of physicians most likely to leave: male, recently completed residency, inexperienced with private practice, and entrepreneurial in spirit. The conclusion was that these individuals tended to leave in favor of situations that afforded them more operational control and gave the perception of opportunity for larger annual increases in compensation. Ongoing recruitment efforts, led by the new chair of family practice, were adjusted to focus more on individuals who had private practice experience and perceived a salaried arrangement as better suited to their needs.

By 1990, when the East Center had been open three years and the North Center two, family practice patient volumes at each center had grown to about 1,000 patients per month. New patients continued to enter the practice at a rate of approximately 300 per center per month. However, a heavy period of turnover struck again in July 1991, and volumes remained relatively flat until July 1992, when full staffing (expanded to five physician FTEs per center) was achieved. Retention of family medicine physicians, which remains a priority challenge, is discussed further in the section on physician compensation.

Family Practice Leadership

The first chairman of family practice had been recruited to Pittsburgh from the Midwest and, as already mentioned, had no relationships within the community or with the local family practice programs. For a variety of reasons, this individual resigned prior to the opening of the first center. The second chair arrived in February 1987 and had contributed significantly to full staffing of both centers by the time the North Center opened. Unfortunately, this physician also resigned, and once again the fledgling program was without leadership.

Chairman turnover, as well as turnover within the ranks of the family practice staff, became the overriding concern of the centers' management team. A search committee was established to study why turnover rates were so high before recruitment of the third—and, hopefully, a long-term—department leader got under way.

Given continued resistance to family practice within the department of medicine, as well as the history of limited chair tenure, recruitment was difficult. The goal was to hire an individual whose credentials were above question, whose interpersonal skills would contribute to improved internal relations with the medical staff, and whose commitment to remaining in the Pittsburgh area was clear.

The third search led to the successful recruitment in fall 1988 of a person who today as chairman of family practice and medical director of the Mercy Family Health Centers continues to meet qualifications. Over time, his commitment to establishing a credible rapport within the department, his integrity and professionalism, and his regular and ongoing efforts to highlight the positive impact of the centers on all facets of the Mercy organization fueled growth in support and appreciation for the benefits provided by the centers. A key contribution was his initiative to make it contractually binding that all physicians who work in the Mercy Family Health Centers be board certified.

175

Physician Compensation

The initial physician contracts provided base salaries ranging from $70,000 to $80,000 per year. This range was determined by a survey of salaries in HMO settings, because the Mercy HMO was the original impetus for development of the centers. Salaries incorporated an incentive component that permitted the medical staff to earn additional income based on patient collections. This incentive was eventually eliminated for legal reasons and because of administrative complexities. Specifically, tracking reimbursement from center physicians' activities under Mercy's accounting system precluded accurate determination of individual physician collections.

By the third year of operation, the family practice contracts became straight-salary arrangements between the hospital and individual physicians. Each physician also could supplement this income by billing independently for his or her inpatient admissions. The opportunity for increases came through annual merit increases based on performance and market adjustments, thus ensuring that base salaries remained competitive with overall market pay. A sample physician performance evaluation form is shown in figure 10-2.

Mercy has monitored national statistics on family medicine compensation, as well as continually updated information on physician salaries in the Pittsburgh area. The current base salary is in the $95,000 to $110,000 range, reflecting increasing competition, both locally and nationally, to employ family medicine physicians. The practice of compensating physicians primarily on a base salary is under review for two reasons: it is believed to contribute to physician turnover by failing to satisfy a need for higher income levels based on performance, and it is suspected to be counterproductive to achieving the centers' desired productivity goals.

Specialty and Support Services

The initial vision and design of the family health centers included additional space for offices and examination rooms intended for time-share rental to specialists who might see patients referred from the family practice or from the local community. The board-approved projections assumed that such tenants would enter the facility simultaneously with the initiation of the primary care practice. Tenant physicians would register and bill their own patients, with the hospital providing space, supplies, reception, and support staff as needed.

In fact it took several years for the rental aspect of the program to fall into place because a number of trial-and-error approaches to allocating and charging for the rental space were applied over the first couple of years. Each approach experimented with varying degrees of flexibility and a range of methods for determining rental fee. Currently, a flat rate per square foot plus additional staff, supplies, and equipment at cost are charged to specialists. However, the most significant issue that seemed to affect the rental program was the success of the primary care practice. As the practice grew and more referrals were directed away from the family medicine program, more specialists chose to add this alternative site to their practices.

During the early years of the centers' operations, experimentation occurred with renting space to non-Mercy care providers. However, over time, enough demand has been generated within the Mercy organization so that only Mercy physicians or programs have been accommodated since 1991. Table 10-2 shows the 1993 service mix at the two centers.

HMO Participation

Concurrent with the planning and implementation of the family health centers, Mercy Hospital's MeSH (Mercy Health United) was busy with development of The HMO Alliance. The HMO product was fully conceptualized, developed, and implemented but was sold within two years of initiation. Early into the experience, Mercy leaders determined that because of the competition in the managed care market and the hospital's limited experience in the insurance business, divestiture of this venture was the most appropriate action.

☐ Outcomes

The four strategic planning objectives referred to earlier in the chapter have met with positive outcomes for the Mercy Family Health Centers. The list on page 178 summarizes these objectives and outcomes.

Figure 10-2. Family Health Centers Performance Evaluation

Physician Name: _____

Date of Evaluation: _____ Rater: _____

	1 = Poor			5 = Excellent	
1. *Departmental functions*					
(a) Attendance and activity at department meetings	1	2	3	4	5
(b) Attendance at committee meetings	1	2	3	4	5
(c) Inpatient activity					
Number	1	2	3	4	5
LOS	1	2	3	4	5
Record-keeping function	1	2	3	4	5
Ability to use the system well	1	2	3	4	5
(d) Other hospital citizenship activity	1	2	3	4	5
2. *Mercy Family Health Center Functions*					
(a) Punctuality	1	2	3	4	5
(b) Medical records functions					
Timeliness	1	2	3	4	5
Completeness	1	2	3	4	5
Conciseness	1	2	3	4	5
Follow-up	1	2	3	4	5
(c) Citizenship					
Staff meeting attendance and activity	1	2	3	4	5
Involvement in center activity	1	2	3	4	5
Center manager relationship	1	2	3	4	5
Medical director relationship	1	2	3	4	5
Relationship with support staff	1	2	3	4	5
(d) Productivity					
Patient volume	1	2	3	4	5
Urgi-care versus family practice attitude	1	2	3	4	5
Ability to hold new patients	1	2	3	4	5
Skill with difficult patients	1	2	3	4	5
Time management skills	1	2	3	4	5
Follow-up of ill patients	1	2	3	4	5
Patient complaints and comments	1	2	3	4	5
Ability with procedural medicine	1	2	3	4	5
Completeness of medical histories	1	2	3	4	5
3. *Personal characteristics*					
(a) Flexibility	1	2	3	4	5
(b) Working as a team member	1	2	3	4	5
(c) Enthusiasm	1	2	3	4	5
(d) Mood	1	2	3	4	5
(e) Maturity	1	2	3	4	5
(f) Stability	1	2	3	4	5
(g) Acceptance of criticism	1	2	3	4	5
(h) Acceptance of direction	1	2	3	4	5

4. *Narrative* _____

_____

_____

Table 10-2. Family Health Centers 1993 Service Mix

Program Services	East	North	Rent Paid
Physician Specialties			
Family practice	X	X	No
Internal medicine		X	Yes
Pediatrics		X	Yes
Ophthalmology	X	X	Yes
General surgery	X	X	Yes
Gastrointestinal surgery	X	X	Yes
Cardiology	X	X	Yes
Psychiatry		X	Yes
Obstetrics/gynecology		X	Yes
Plastic surgery	X	X	Yes
Ancillaries			
Basic laboratory	X	X	No
Basic radiology	X	X	No
Mammography		X	No
Physical therapy	X	X	No
Other Hospital Services			
Cancer screening	X	X	No
National Heart Attack Risk Study	X	X	No
Natural family planning classes	X	X	No
Drug and alcohol counseling		X	Yes
Nutrition counseling	X	X	No

1. *Primary care referral base linked to Mercy's specialty and subspecialty services:* The bar chart in figure 10-3 illustrates the referral patterns from the centers. Referred fee-for-service inpatient admissions to Mercy Hospital, although growing, have been one of the more disappointing areas. Original performance projections assumed 1–3 percent of visits would result in admissions to the hospital; however, the actual rate is less than 1 percent. Referrals to Mercy specialists and ancillary departments continue to grow and are regarded as a strong positive feature.

2. *Geographic distribution of Mercy health care services/entry into the Mercy System:* The family health centers are regarded as Mercy's service delivery points north and east of Pittsburgh. Although HMO growth in Pittsburgh has been steady since the early 1980s, there was never a period of rapid growth, and as of 1993 managed care remains at less than 20 percent of the total insurance market. However, current events foretell a significant and rapid surge in this percentage. Center practices are regarded as key components to Mercy's successful positioning for this conversion.

   In addition, in 1993 The Pittsburgh Mercy Health System acquired a second acute care facility located on the north side of Pittsburgh. It is expected that admissions from this center will improve, as the facility is closer to and more accessible for both patients and medical staff.

3. *Elimination of gaps in the HMO delivery and service network:* With the sale of the Mercy HMO shortly after the centers opened, this objective became less of a priority in the early years of center development. However, as discussed above, the centers are seen as important elements of Mercy's current positioning for success in a managed care environment in that they provide key linkages in The Pittsburgh Mercy Health System's primary care network.

4. *Creation of an environment that will foster evolution of a multispecialty group practice at Mercy:* Although a formal multispecialty group practice has not yet developed at Mercy, market conditions have prompted real progress toward this goal in the

Figure 10-3. Family Health Centers Referral History

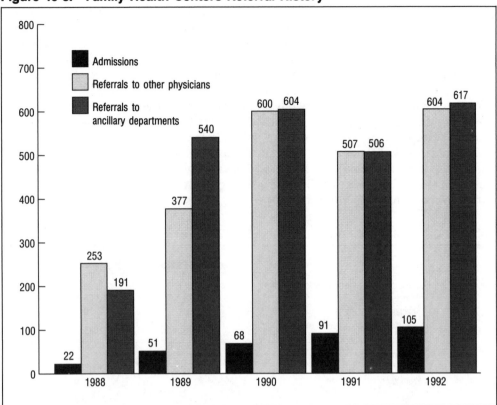

near future. The centers are recognized as potential worksites for the planned multi-specialty service.

Aside from specific attainments in terms of the original goals, positive outcomes have been achieved in other critical areas as well. Financial growth, operational evolution, special program development, and changes in the family practice component are a few outcomes described briefly in the following sections.

Financial Results

After five years of operation, each center's volume of family practice visits reached approximately 16,000 (1993 results). Although the centers continue to demonstrate growth and growth potential, actual performance has differed from original assumptions that from their inception the centers would behave like mature family practices. The reality is that the early practice looked more like an urgi-care center than a mature practice. This has changed, and in 1993 in excess of 80 percent of center activity was due to patients returning for care.

Changes in payer mix are expected beginning in 1994, with a continuing shift toward increased workers' compensation cases and managed care. Blue Cross and commercial insurance volumes are declining. Mercy Hospital maintains a philosophy of a preferential option for the medically indigent, as demonstrated by a growing percentage of Medicaid patients at both centers. This portion of the centers' activity is also expected to increase slightly as Mercy becomes involved in a Medicaid HMO.

Conducting financial analyses is a challenging task due to limitations in the hospital's outpatient information systems and billing practices. Consequently, attempts to relate patient care receipts to direct operating expenses must be based on billing audits and assumptions. Furthermore, other hospital departments utilize center space for their programs without paying rent, although center staff and resources provide registration, telephone, and waiting room support services. For accounting purposes, patient revenues and volumes for these programs accrue to the respective department. In addition, although the centers' laboratories provide a limited set of on-site testing, the majority of specimens are transported to the main laboratory on the hospital campus. Revenues for these tests accrue to the main lab, not to the family centers. Finally, each year the centers refer hundreds of patients out of the facilities to other Mercy Hospital departments, medical staff practices, or to the acute facility for admission. Revenues for these referrals (except for the admissions) are very difficult to track.

Despite the limitations cited, direct profit and loss analyses are conducted for each center each year. (See tables 10-3 and 10-4.) These analyses continue to show losses from direct operations. However, the benefits accruing to the rest of the organization are estimated to more than offset the direct operating losses.

Table 10-3. Profit and Loss Summary, East Center

	Two Years Previous	Previous Year
Number of full-time-equivalent physicians		
Primary care	3.25	3.25
Specialists	0	0
Total	3.25	3.25
Collections		
Fee for service	$779,753	$761,593
Prepaid	0	0
Total	$779,753	$761,593
Expenses		
Operations	$625,203	$637,867
Physicians[a]	$317,788	$324,942
Total	$942,991	$962,809
Surplus (deficit)	($163,238)	($201,216)

[a]Includes physician salaries and benefits.

Table 10-4. Profit and Loss Summary, North Center

	Two Years Previous	Previous Year
Number of full-time-equivalent physicians		
Primary care	3.66	3.66
Specialists	0	0
Total	3.66	3.66
Collections		
Fee for service	$793,089	$827,460
Prepaid	0	0
Total	$793,089	$827,460
Expenses		
Operations	$631,091	$637,842
Physicians[a]	$270,468	$275,692
Total	$901,559	$913,534
Surplus (deficit)	($108,470)	($ 86,074)

[a]Includes physician salaries and benefits.

Operational Issues

The choice to set up the centers as extensions of the hospital outpatient program has created some challenges for routine center operations. Billing is done by the hospital through Medicare Part A and Blue Cross. Under the cost-based method of payment, it is difficult to monitor actual patient receipts on a center-by-center, case-by-case basis. As a result, center managers have difficulty monitoring direct operating performance.

At the patient service level, this arrangement has also created some challenges. For example, under a system of electronic patient registration, the centers transmit registration information by modem to the finance department staff, located at the main hospital campus, who generate the bill. Initially center staff were unfamiliar with the billing process because it was not part of their responsibilities. Eventually, customer service problems arose when a patient contacted a center with billing questions that center staff could not answer because they had not initiated the bill. This problem was addressed by training the center support staff in hospital billing procedures and by making the billing record accessible electronically to the centers.

Other operational issues arise as center managers work to coordinate the variety of other hospital programs and medical staff who use the center as a site for their service delivery. Planning, organization, and communications skills are constantly in demand to ensure scheduling that enables successful program implementation and growth without adversely affecting the family practice operations. The following discussion addresses the range of services currently facilitated through use of center space.

Specialty Program Development

Although early demand for space in the family centers was slow in developing, current growth is steady. The range of services offered through the two centers was discussed earlier and is detailed in table 10-2.

An unexpected area of growth for the Family Health Centers has been the number of other Mercy departments that use the centers as "outlets" for their programs. For example, Mercy's physical therapy, nutrition counseling, and mental health counseling services are now available at both centers. In addition, the Mercy Heart Institute uses the centers as screening sites for patients participating in the National Heart Attack Risk Study. Similarly, the Mercy Cancer Center conducts cancer screenings in these facilities. A particularly good growth area since 1991 has been occupational health services, marketed through the hospital's HealthForce program. Mercy Hospital–based programs using the family health centers as distribution sites for their services are not charged rent for the space, a practice that exacerbates difficulties in determining actual financial performance of the centers.

Family Practice Issues

July 1992 was the first time since 1989 that all family practice contracts were renewed for another year. However, one physician left in July 1993, and the recruitment process was reinitiated. Compensation continues to be a key negotiation issue as family practitioners experience high demand in a low-supply market.

Organizing family practice physicians into an independent practice plan that contracts with the hospital to provide medical services in the centers remains an option. The goal of a revised structure will be to improve overall financial performance of the centers from the hospital's viewpoint, while providing incentives for physicians to increase productivity as monitored against predetermined quality and performance standards. The revised structure is intended to give the physicians a greater sense of ownership, commitment, and opportunity for financial benefit than is available in a full-salary arrangement. However, efforts to pursue this option are not active at this time.

☐ **Future Outlook**

The Mercy Family Health Centers have been a challenging opportunity to establish hospital-owned primary care practices in locations not previously served by the institution. The decision to sell The HMO Alliance in 1988 removed one of the primary objectives originally set to develop the centers. However, having formal linkages with a geographically distributed primary care network continues to be a strategic requirement of the hospital as it expands participation in managed care arrangements; so the centers continue to provide a strategic benefit to the organization.

As Mercy plans further development of its primary care program, the following lessons learned from the Family Health Centers will be helpful to remember:

- The time frame needed to establish a new primary care practice with physicians who have no practice history in the target area is lengthy. Acquiring or linking with existing practices would permit quicker market entry with less financial risk.
- Physicians with subspecialty practices require a referral pool with proved potential before they consider entering a new geographic area.
- Many existing hospital outpatient information systems are inadequate for monitoring the direct financial performance of a hospital-based center. Similarly, hospital-based billing staffs tend to be more inpatient oriented than outpatient oriented. Customer service and management accountability would be improved with center-based independent, but integrated, billing systems.
- It is difficult to justify the development of a freestanding, hospital-owned primary care center on its direct financial performance from operations. The facility should have demonstrable strategic benefit as identified specifically in the context of a hospital strategic plan.
- Family practice physicians are currently in high demand. Consequently, the risk of turnover is high, and compensation packages are growing at a faster rate than those for other physician specialties. Potential employers of primary care physicians must understand their income needs. Furthermore, recruiters must balance these needs with the candidates' lifestyle requirements (such as a predictable work schedule and limited call duty).

The Mercy Hospital of Pittsburgh intends to further develop its primary care network. However, future approaches are less likely to include attempts to build new practices from scratch. Because they have become established practices, the two Mercy family health centers will serve as core sites for the development of an expanded array of hospital programs and services. Additional locations are likely to be developed around existing practices in target communities, in collaboration with established primary care physicians who wish to affiliate with the hospital.

Chapter 11

St. Luke's Hospital

Spencer Maidlow, President and CEO,
and Nancy Graebner, Director of Medical Practices,
St. Luke's Hospital, Saginaw, MI

☐ Executive Summary: Key Elements of the Affiliation

- *Organizational structure:* A hospital establishes a hospital-owned OB/GYN group practice and employs three physicians. Management for the practice and supervision of the physicians is provided through the medical affairs department of the hospital, which operates this practice and other practices owned by the hospital.
- *Hospital goals:* The hospital had responded to the needs of several staff physicians in acquiring and managing their practices and then employing the physicians. As part of the hospital's strategy to meet community need and expand its services to meet the demands of managed care contracting, the hospital developed maternity services and established a new OB/GYN group practice.
- *Physician needs and goals:* Staff physicians sought hospital support in meeting the financial needs of their practices in response to reduced reimbursement and demands of managed care contracts. The physicians were also supportive of the hospital's goals to expand services to contract effectively with managed care providers.
- *Personal relationships:* Through formal and informal communication with the medical staff, the hospital had built a high level of trust with the physicians. Hospital management was respected by the physicians and there was little doubt that the hospital's goals and objectives were compatible with the physicians' needs.
- *Health care reform and managed care:* St. Luke's market had not experienced significant impact from health care reform or the introduction of insurance products that reimbursed physicians on a capitated basis. However, insurance companies were developing exclusive panels of providers to control utilization of care given to their enrollees, and increased risk-sharing contracts throughout Michigan were anticipated to affect the Saginaw market.
- *Capital needs and resources:* St. Luke's Hospital had established a budget for practice acquisition and start-up, as well as a staff to provide management services to physician practices, as a result of its acquisition of practices over a period of several years. Capital was required to renovate the hospital so as to provide maternity services and to acquire the equipment and furnishing needed for an OB/GYN

practice. Based on the medical staff development plan, the hospital also had a budget for physician recruitment.

- *Physician recruitment and retention:* Recruitment of OB/GYN physicians was difficult due to strong competition for the specialty nationwide. An attractive employment package was developed, and emphasis was placed on identifying candidates who shared the philosophy and approach to providing maternity services established at the hospital and its practice.

- *Legal and contracting issues:* St. Luke's went through a lengthy certificate-of-need process to obtain authorization to develop maternity services. Physician employment contracts had been developed in the past and were modified to meet the needs of OB/GYN physicians. Community needs assessment and documentation to justify physician income under the employment agreement were completed to comply with legal and regulatory issues relating to private inurement and Medicare fraud and abuse.

☐ Introduction

The decision to introduce maternity services at St. Luke's Hospital in Saginaw, Michigan, in 1989 created an immediate need for OB/GYN physicians. Because St. Luke's owned and operated several medical practices, it was able to start a hospital-owned OB/GYN practice that has grown into a three-physician group in less than three years. By 1993, deliveries in the new maternity unit had grown from 0 to more than 600, and the OB/GYN practice was projected to break even in 1994.

☐ Background

Saginaw is located halfway up the southern peninsula of Michigan. Traditionally, its economy depended on manufacturing, agriculture, higher education, and health care. Over the past 10 years, employment at the area's five major General Motors facilities has fallen by 30 percent. Efforts made by Saginaw hospitals to expand services to a larger geographic area, coupled with expanding employment in small businesses and industries in the community, have promoted growth in the health care segment of the city's economy.

St. Luke's Hospital is a 352-bed, not-for-profit general medical and surgical facility founded in 1887. St. Luke's participates in four residency programs (family practice, OB/GYN, internal medicine, and general surgery) with the other two hospitals in Saginaw. Its primary service area is populated by approximately 221,000 residents. The referral service area comprises 800,000 people. Of the two other general medical and surgical facilities in Saginaw, one has 309 beds and the other has 268 beds.

Approximately 25 percent of St. Luke's service area is enrolled in managed care programs with minimal capitated products. Only 5 percent of St. Luke's inpatient business is managed care, reflecting the health care status of the population covered by managed care and the physicians' discipline in treating managed care patients outside the hospital.

The city's medical community consists mostly of solo or small single-specialty group practices. The physicians have maintained independence from the hospitals and third-party payers, maintaining privileges at all three area hospitals and participating in managed care on a selective, contract-by-contract basis. There are 323 physicians on St. Luke's medical staff.

The three area hospitals have pursued a strategy of "cooperative competition" throughout their history. More than 20 joint ventures among them exist in the form of residency training, helipads, laboratory services, and ambulatory facilities. As recently as 1971, all maternity care in Saginaw was performed at Saginaw General Hospital. The other two hospitals, including St. Luke's, dropped their obstetrical services, with the exception of a few deliveries at a 171-bed osteopathic hospital with 14 licensed obstetrical beds.

Hospital

In 1986 St. Luke's developed a service expansion strategy, a major component of which was obstetrical (OB) services. This decision was reached as a result of the following influences:

- *Managed care demands:* The market penetration by managed care programs created a consumer demand for full-service contracts from providers.
- *Competition:* Competitor hospitals began to expand services, develop formal affiliations with physician practices, and penetrate new market areas.
- *Identified community need for obstetric services:* A 1983 study ("Health Systems Plan") conducted by the East Central Michigan Health Systems Agency (HSA) for the Saginaw Health Service Area confirmed the need for all 69 licensed OB beds, including those at Saginaw General and the 14 beds at the osteopathic hospital. Market studies demonstrated that more than 1,000 patients from the primary service area utilized institutions outside the HSA for their obstetrical care. This represented nearly 25 percent of the area's total obstetrical caseload in 1986. Surveys concluded that the two reasons for this out-migration were:
  - High census of existing HSA obstetrical beds
  - Absence of a labor, delivery, recovery, and postpartum (LDRP) unit in the HSA institutions

In 1987 St. Luke's purchased the 171-bed osteopathic hospital—including the 14 licensed maternity beds—as part of its strategic plan, primarily to expand inpatient and outpatient psychiatric services.

Medical Staff Relationship

St. Luke's board and administration had developed a good relationship with the medical staff through open communication, effective involvement of the medical staff leadership in the hospital's decision-making process, and concerted efforts to resolve issues raised by the medical staff. Furthermore, medical staff participation on the board and board committees was encouraged. The CEO and the vice-president for medical affairs (a position created in 1988 and filled with a well-respected, local family medicine physician) hold monthly dinner meetings with the officers of the medical staff. At these meetings, the hospital's strategic initiatives are discussed, and the medical staff leaders provide input.

Medical staff officers are also invited to participate in quarterly strategic retreat/dinner meetings with members of the board so as to focus on single issues and arrive at strategic direction. Topics have included analysis and reaction to new outpatient facilities at St. Luke's, the 20-year facilities master plan, St. Luke's transition to a total quality management culture, development of a "Preferred Future" (strategies for approaching managed care), and the role of the board and medical leaders in institutional leadership. Additionally, medical staff leaders are invited to attend the board's annual planning retreat and all its social events.

☐ Hospital Practice Acquisition and Development

This section recounts the activities that led to the hospital's acquisition and development of physician practices. The first informal discussion that became the catalyst for hospital ownership is described. Additionally, practice valuation, management operations, and the development of physician employment contracts and compensation packages are discussed.

Initiation of Practice Acquisitions

St. Luke's first became involved in the ownership of physician practices in 1988, when a solo family practitioner requested that the hospital purchase his practice and employ him in the practice. This request was in reaction to two factors: the increasing administrative burdens of operating a practice, and the fact that the other hospitals in Saginaw were purchasing medical practices. Pursuant to discussions among the hospital's board of directors, medical staff leaders, and administrators, St. Luke's made the purchase but limited its future involvement in practice acquisition in the following ways:

- Existing practices would be purchased only at the request of their physician owners.
- Medical practices would receive hospital support only after a determination that specific community needs were being satisfied.
- St. Luke's would initiate new practices only in specialties identified by the board, medical staff leadership, and management as being needed in the community, and where no private practice alternatives for the recruitment of these specialists exists.

Subject to these three conditions, eight practices were purchased between 1988 and 1990: four existing solo family medicine practices, a two-physician internal medicine group, a psychiatric practice, and two urgi-care centers. In addition, based on community needs assessment and strategic planning, St. Luke's recruited physicians and developed hospital-owned practices in pediatric surgery, pediatric intensive care, anesthesia, child psychiatry, and neurosurgery. Although the medical staff has supported these efforts and worked well with the physicians employed by the hospital, staff members continue to favor independence from the hospital.

Financial issues that received much attention in the purchasing process included practice valuation, physician salary and incentives, and a noncompete clause prohibiting physicians from leaving and establishing a new practice within 30 miles of the existing practice until three years after the separation date. Responsibility for the overall purchase, setup, and operation of the practices (with the exception of the hospital-based specialist practices) rests with the vice-president for medical affairs and the director of medical practice management.

Practice Valuation

Practice purchases initially were based on individual negotiations with physician owners. An overall value was determined based on a percentage of gross practice charges during the year immediately preceding the purchase. The value assigned using this approach and the negotiation process was derived from hard assets, practice goodwill, and a noncompete agreement (if applicable). Future practice purchases are anticipated to be based on hard asset value only, unless physician owners anticipate retirement within one year. This change in approach was made so that St. Luke's could remain in compliance with antifraud laws and safe harbors. Also, based on opinion from legal counsel that its enforcement would be difficult, the hospital eliminated the noncompete agreement.

Accounts receivable prior to purchase date were retained by the physician and not considered in the purchase. In one case real estate was purchased, but the rest of the practices remain in rental space, a decision based on the large capital requirements of real estate purchase and on the long-term inflexibility of real estate ownership.

Practice Management

A medical practice management department was established under the medical affairs division for the purpose of operating hospital-owned practices. (See figures 11-1 and 11-2.) In creating this department, the hospital relied on the experience of the vice-president for medical affairs, who previously owned a successful family practice, and the department

Figure 11-1. Hospital Organizational Flowchart

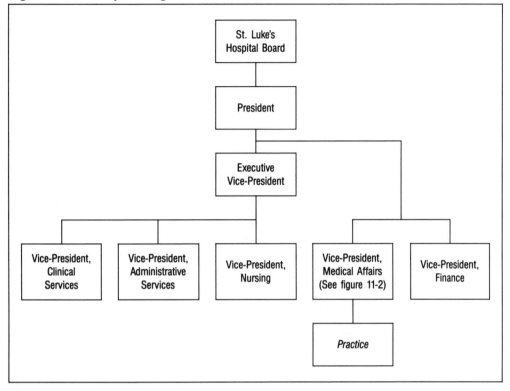

director, who had eight years of practice management experience (including physician billing and coding). Backed by this depth of experience on the part of key personnel, St. Luke's was able to quickly develop the ability to evaluate practice operations, verify valuations, and set up effective systems within the acquired practices.

Each practice has a designated office manager who oversees day-to-day operations; the physician has responsibility for the clinical aspects of the practice. Purchasing, accounting, budgeting, staffing and human resource functions, and marketing are centralized through the medical practice management department. The physician has certain input into operational issues such as employee selection, equipment purchases, marketing, and so forth. Billing and collections are handled independently at each practice site, under the direction of the department, and use the standing practice billing system or, if replacement or start-up is in order, a system selected by the department.

All practice employees are hired through the medical practice department. Candidates are screened by the office manager and then interviewed by the physicians who will work with them in the practice. Final selection is based on mutual agreement. Salary levels and benefits are set at the low end of the hospital ranges because the job descriptions differ from those in acute care settings and, unlike acute care settings, there is no shift or weekend work. Also, salaries and benefits are set in line with the physician office marketplace.

A budget is developed for each practice that includes a management fee (typically between $2,000 and $5,000 per year). Applicable amortization of the practice purchase price is included in the overhead expense calculations of the hospital-owned practices.

Physician Employment

All physicians in the hospital-owned practices are employed by the hospital, with base salaries and incentive bonuses based on practice operation results and market standards.

Figure 11-2. Medical Affairs Division Organizational Flowchart

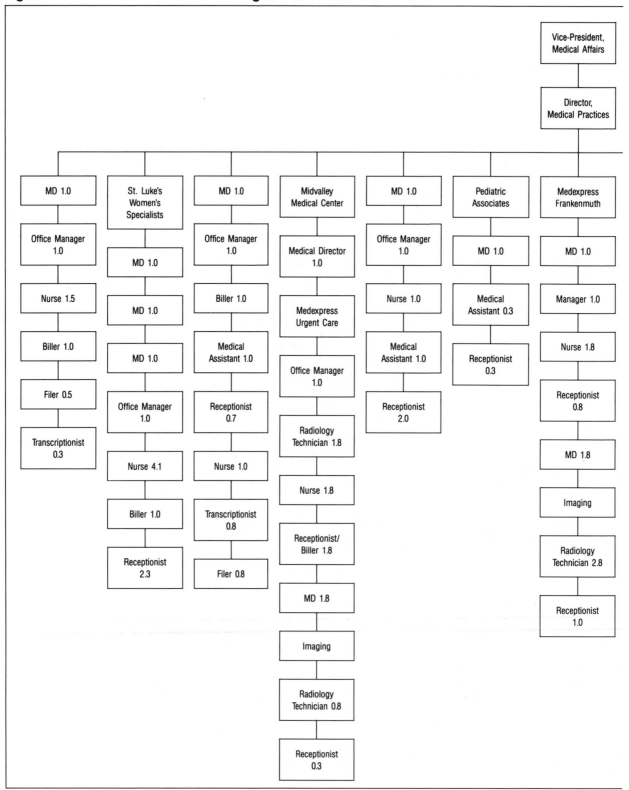

Note: The numbers listed after each position represent the number of full-time equivalents based on 2,080 hours per year.

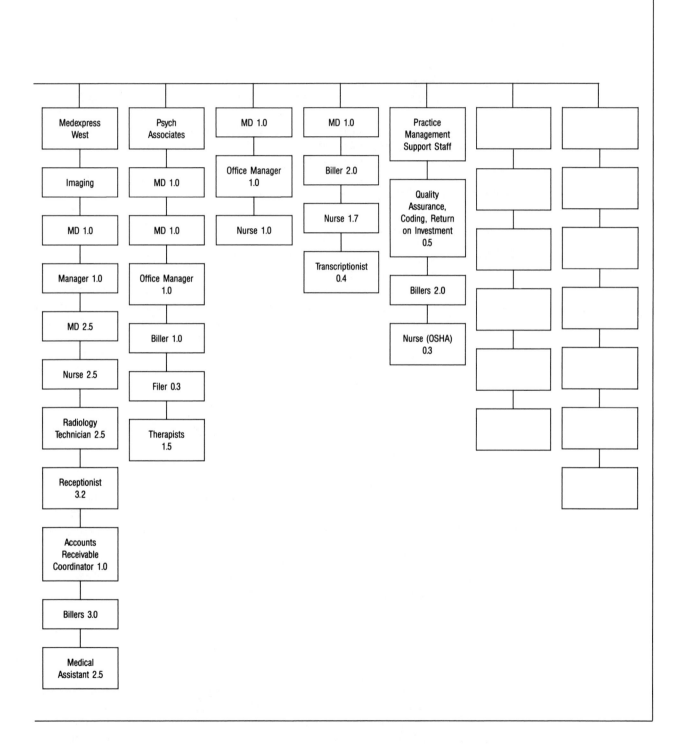

Although Michigan has a corporate practice of medicine statute, it has not been enforced and is currently under review by the attorney general as to whether it will remain on the books. St. Luke's Hospital elected to proceed with this approach based on the similar activities of other hospitals in Michigan and after consultation with hospital legal counsel.

The initial employment contracts were customized to each physician, for both existing practices and new practices established for needed specialties. This lack of uniformity created more problems than it solved. Various changes in the hospital's relationship with the practices required intensive review of each contract. As a result, a model contract has been developed that serves as the starting point for negotiations. Deviations from the model must be cleared with the vice-president of medical affairs before finalization. The original contracts have been renegotiated to comply with the terms of the new contract.

Two key areas are emphasized in discussions with physicians who seek employment with the hospital. One involves authority and responsibility parameters for practice operations as described earlier. The other deals with productivity expectations of the practice and the relationship between practice net revenues and the incentive component of the physician compensation package.

Physician Compensation

In determining a base salary for physicians in existing practices, the mean of the physician's past three years' net income (determined from income tax returns) is projected forward. That figure is then evaluated in light of what similar specialists earn, nationally and locally. In the case of new residents, salary is based on the average income for that specialty, with consideration given to the physician's current financial circumstances. Ultimately, negotiations with the physician lead to an agreement on the base salary.

Incentives include the first several thousand dollars of net income generated over and above the practice expenses. For this formula, practice overhead expenses include the physician's base salary, malpractice insurance, and cost of benefits. Additional profit above the first several thousand dollars is split 50–50 between the physician and St. Luke's.

☐ The New OB/GYN Practice

St. Luke's approach to determining physician recruitment priorities and whether to establish a hospital-sponsored practice is comprehensive and involves key members of the medical staff. Research findings concluded that the service area was in need of OB/GYN specialists. Despite this fact, the medical staff had mixed reactions to the plan for a new family-oriented obstetrical program at St. Luke's.

Supported by community needs assessment, market expansion, and hospital service initiatives, St. Luke's developed a comprehensive physician manpower plan. Specific recommendations were presented to the medical staff leadership by the vice-president for medical affairs, with supporting data that previously were reviewed by the administration and the board.

Group Practice

St. Luke's documented a need for 25 OB/GYN specialists in the service area, 8 more than the current number. In addition, the reaction on the part of OB/GYN physicians in the community to the hospital's development of maternity services (described in the following section) was further support that active OB/GYN physicians were needed on St. Luke's medical staff. The process established earlier for initiating hospital-owned practices, as well as the resources and procedures already developed for managing practices and employing physicians, allowed St. Luke's to quickly draw up and approve a plan to create a hospital-owned OB/GYN practice to meet these needs.

Reactions to the Plan

Discussions with the medical staff concerning the introduction of a new, family-oriented obstetrical program at St. Luke's received mixed reactions. Most staff, including family medicine physicians also involved in obstetrics, supported the program. Discussions with family medicine physicians indicated that a large percentage of their patient base wanted a family-oriented maternity service. Their having selected a family medicine practitioner over an OB/GYN specialist was partly attributable to their interest in family-oriented maternity care.

St. Luke's active medical staff included 12 OB/GYN specialists at the time this plan was originated. Their hospital activity was limited to GYN surgery, because the majority of their inpatient activity occurred at a hospital that had OB facilities. Only one of these specialists supported St. Luke's new program; the remaining 11 cited the following objections:

- Inability of a number of Saginaw hospitals to support maternity services in the past
- Concern for patient care in a hospital ill equipped to handle severe obstetrical and neonatal complications
- Scheduling conflicts that precluded the current OB/GYN physicians from providing sufficient maternity coverage at two hospitals, given the large number of deliveries in their existing practices

Upon approval in 1988 to open the new OB service at St. Luke's, 11 of the hospital's 12 specialists withdrew from the medical staff in protest. To date, they have not sought to reinstate their staff privileges.

The hospital's position was that the potential success of its overall plan took precedence over the loss of GYN volume attributable to the departing OB/GYN physicians. To move forward with the development of a maternity service, the medical affairs division was charged with recruiting physicians and establishing a hospital-owned OB/GYN practice.

☐ Implementation

The implementation effort involved a number of tasks, not least of which was immediate recruitment of OB/GYN physicians. Also, an employment package had to be developed, as well as a marketing campaign to announce the service. Once the service was implemented, rapid growth had to be addressed. Details of these implementation issues are related in the following sections.

Physician Recruitment and Employment

As anticipated, the recruitment of OB/GYN physicians was complicated because of the high demand for this specialty nationwide. Furthermore, state and local market conditions and competitor activity meant that candidates would have to be offered an aggressive compensation package. For example, malpractice insurance expense alone for OB/GYN physicians was higher in Michigan than in most other states, with annual costs exceeding $55,000. An additional concern was whether the appeal to relocate to Saginaw, Michigan, would be strong enough for candidates, given the economy, climate, and competition from more cosmopolitan urban centers.

Working with the board of directors and medical staff leadership, the hospital determined that recruitment efforts should center on physicians who wanted to work in an

OB/GYN practice that emphasizes family-oriented OB care. This strategy, along with a good compensation package, on-call coverage from other physicians, and the security of hospital employment would be an optimal package to attract new OB/GYN physicians.

After an 18-month search that involved several recruiting firms, a candidate was identified in early 1990. Although currently in practice with a group elsewhere in Michigan, he was eager to find a location in which he could pursue his interest in family-oriented obstetrical care. The physician's motivations appeared compatible with those of the hospital.

After several visits to Saginaw, the candidate agreed to employment at St. Luke's, effective August 1990. Admitting privileges for the candidate were pursued at Saginaw General for provision of delivery services during completion of the St. Luke's facility. Initially, Saginaw's OB/GYN staff challenged this privilege, and an offer was issued for him to join an existing OB/GYN group on Saginaw General Hospital's staff. Both efforts were unsuccessful, and St. Luke's initial recruitment effort with the candidate was realized.

Specific details of the employment offer are confidential, but compensation included a salary in excess of $180,000, an incentive package based on practice revenues, and full benefits including malpractice insurance. Because St. Luke's is self-insured for malpractice coverage, the actual cost was not as high as statewide figures. St. Luke's continued offering attractive incentives in negotiations to expand the OB/GYN practice.

Practice volume grew quickly (as detailed later in this chapter), and a second OB/GYN physician joined the practice in July 1991. This individual was recruited from the community's OB residency program, and the process proved easier this time around. The combination of practice appeal and inpatient service again were coupled with an attractive compensation package. However, the second physician resigned from the practice in August 1992, electing instead to pursue missionary work.

Patient survey results had reflected a community desire for female OB/GYN physicians. Through a fortunate set of circumstances, accommodating this demand proved to be relatively easy. One woman was chief resident in the hospitals' OB residency program. Another was the wife of an oncologist who was relocating to the area; she also was recruited as faculty to the residency program. A growing OB practice that was affiliated with a family-oriented delivery service appealed to both new recruits.

Marketing the OB/GYN Practice

St. Luke's marketing efforts focused on the family-oriented approach to the OB services offered in its new practice, capitalizing on the fact that the maternity facility a physician uses is likely to influence a patient's choice of physician. The hospital also recognized that existing OB physicians in the Saginaw area were not interested in using St. Luke's new facility. Therefore, marketing efforts included news releases, patient newsletters, and brochures emphasizing the new physician's focus on family-oriented OB care and specifically the new maternity services at St. Luke's. In late 1990, consumer surveys indicated a 45 percent awareness level of the new services after one month of marketing effort.

☐ Practice Results

The development of the OB/GYN practice involved significant investments. Initially, St. Luke's did not develop time frames to achieve practice volumes that would ensure break-even status. However, St. Luke's board of directors recognized the importance of family-oriented OB services in the community and that the OB/GYN practice would be instrumental to the IP unit's success. To help ensure the success of the practice, St. Luke's made its customary practice expectations known and monitored the practice's actual results.

Hospital Expectations

Traditionally, St. Luke's board of directors expects new programs to break even within a three-year period. In the case of the 16 medical practices owned by the hospital, however, no specific return-on-investment targets were set. The objective of purchasing or establishing new medical practices was driven by the board's desire to contribute to the range of services offered to the community. Even so, expectations are that the practices will cover all their operating expenses both from a business investment perspective and to avoid private inurement issues related to the hospital's tax-exempt status. Most of a practice's additional net income, if any, is returned to the physician through a bonus as recognition for productivity.

Because of the significant start-up costs associated with the new OB/GYN practice, primarily in recruitment expenses and salary guarantees, the board was aware that this effort might require a longer investment period. The board also recognized the importance of this practice to implementation of the new inpatient maternity service.

The hospital's experience with transition of existing private practices to hospital-owned status was that a three-year time frame to cover expenses was reasonable in the purchase of existing primary care practices, but the time required for new specialty practices to break even was not as predictable. The emphasis on obstetrics in the new practice affected financial expectations as well. For example, revenues in OB/GYN practices typically include a significant volume of GYN surgery for which no projections were made in the first few years of this new practice.

Practice Volume

Practice growth exceeded expectations. Patient visits increased from 2,875 in the first full year of operation to a projected 14,400 in the fourth year. The number of physicians went from one to three during this same period.

The number of deliveries performed in the OB/GYN practice during the same period grew from 82 to more than 400 projected in year 4. First-year net revenues of $256,000 reached $650,000 and beyond in year 3, with a profit anticipated for year 4. Capital investments for equipment and furnishings were $20,000 in year 1 and $40,000 in year 3, when space was doubled and renovated to accommodate three physicians. Managed care revenue continues to represent less than 15 percent of total revenues, with no capitated contracts at this time. (See table 11-1.)

Maternity Services

Successful growth in the total number of deliveries at St. Luke's has been largely due to the development of the new OB/GYN group practice. The first calendar year saw 430 deliveries,

Table 11-1. OB/GYN Practice Financial Results

	7/1/90 to 6/30/91	7/1/91 to 6/30/92	7/1/92 to 6/3/93
Number of full-time-equivalent physicians:	1	2	2.8
Collections:[a]			
Medicare/Medicaid	$104,867	$159,651	$176,464
Fee for service	99,752	362,285	400,438
Managed care	51,155	92,106	101,806
Total	$255,774	$614,042	$678,708
Expenses:			
Capital investment	$ 20,000		$ 40,000
Operations	113,791	$146,257	146,302
Physicians' compensation and benefits[b]	252,250	474,500	696,750
Total	$386,041	$620,757	$883,052
Surplus (deficit):	($130,267)	($6,715)	($204,344)

[a]Net charges after adjustments.
[b]Does not include malpractice or retirement contribution.

47 percent by OB/GYN physicians and 53 percent by family medicine physicians. In the second calendar year, 630 deliveries were performed, 55 percent by OB/GYN physicians and 45 percent by family medicine physicians.

☐ Outcomes and Lessons Learned

The following conclusions can be drawn from St. Luke's experience in developing a hospital-owned OB/GYN group practice:

- St. Luke's approach to acquiring or establishing physician practices has been accepted among its physicians, despite the medical staff's philosophical preference for autonomy among attending staff. This acceptance was achieved as a result of the hospital's:
  - Communicating openly with medical staff leaders, starting with the initial request by a member of the medical staff for St. Luke's to purchase his practice
  - Establishing and maintaining the position to only purchase existing practices at the physician owner's request *or* to open new specialty practices only where a community need has been documented and agreed to by all parties concerned
  - Providing the necessary management and financial resources to run the practices effectively
- Accurate assessment of community need and patient preference has been demonstrated by the rapid growth of the OB/GYN practice.
- Financial growth and stability of the practice can be attributed in part to the development of a recruitment strategy that recognized not only physicians' financial expectations, but also the need for common goals on the part of management and practice physicians.
- Evolution of in-depth orientation of employed physicians to their role in a hospital-owned and managed practice has clarified mutual expectations.
- St. Luke's conservative approach toward growth of physician practice ownership and management has allowed management adequate time to develop expertise and systems to operate a practice effectively.

☐ Future Outlook

In looking ahead, St Luke's has several goals for its hospital-sponsored OB/GYN practice:

- Increase gynecological surgery services.
- Add a fourth physician as soon as patient volumes can support one.
- Increase the percentage of Medicaid OB services in response to community need.
- Assist with OB coverage for adjoining rural communities.
- Support expansion of the inpatient OB unit (The Family Birth Center).
- Establish satellite OB clinics to enlarge the physician referral base.

Efforts are under way to develop centralized computer billing services for the hospital-owned practices. Strategic plans include expansion of practice management to independent practices on a contract basis; one such contract has been initiated for the management of a three-physician practice.

Another project will be to bring together St. Luke's affiliated practices into a group practice model and introduce additional physician services identified as needed in the Saginaw community. It is anticipated that such a group practice would form an important part of a St. Luke's managed care strategy, involving both employed and independent physicians who will negotiate managed care contracts as a group rather than individually. The medical staff remains wary of the hospital's involvement in physician practices, but because the hospital has maintained a nonaggressive, supportive stance, physicians are more open to discussion and expansion of St. Luke's involvement.

Chapter 12

Monroe Clinic/St. Clare Hospital

Dennis J. Tomczyk, Vice-President, Health Services Development,
James Davidson, MD, and James D. Beyers, President,
Monroe Clinic, Monroe, WI

☐ Executive Summary: Key Elements of the Affiliation

- *Organizational structure:* A hospital acquires an existing multispecialty group practice whose members represent the majority of its medical staff. The physicians are employed by the hospital.
- *Hospital goals:* The Hospital had short-term needs to recruit additional primary care and specialist physicians as well as to ensure the survival of a group practice that dominated its medical staff. The Hospital had identified the long-term strategic goal of developing additional formal affiliations with this practice group in order to move toward an integrated system for the delivery of health care.
- *Physician needs and goals:* The group practice had immediate financial concerns and the physician owners were unable to reach consensus on a strategy to resolve them.
- *Personal relationships:* Leadership changes, both in the Hospital and the group practice, led to improved personal relationships and trust between both entities.
- *Health care reform and managed care:* The Monroe, Wisconsin, market has not been significantly affected by health care reform or the introduction of insurance products that reimburse providers on a capitated basis. Reduced reimbursement from Medicare and the need to provide services to the medically indigent population were important motivations for the affiliation.
- *Market and competitor activities:* The Hospital and group practice were the sole providers for the Monroe service area for most health care services. There was concern over the geographic expansion of competing hospitals and physician groups from surrounding counties, although this threat was not deemed significant.
- *Capital needs and resources:* Capital was needed for the acquisition of the group practice and its integration with the Hospital. Financing for construction of a new clinic facility, major renovations to the Hospital, start-up funds, and practice transition was obtained through issuance of a tax-exempt bond to the Hospital.
- *Physician recruitment and retention:* The financial stability of the Hospital–group practice affiliation enhanced physician recruitment and retention. For example, competitive salaries based on physician productivity could be guaranteed as a result of the affiliation, in contrast to the prior practice of paying physicians out of the money available after practice expenses were met.

- *Legal and contracting issues:* Because of how the Hospital's legal counsel interpreted the laws and regulations related to private inurement and Medicare fraud and abuse, the Hospital elected not to purchase intangible assets of the practice. In acquiring the practice and employing the physicians, St. Clare Hospital circumvented major legal issues.

☐ Introduction

St. Clare Hospital (the Hospital) purchased the Monroe Clinic (the Clinic) in May 1992. Founded in 1939, both organizations flourished through the mid-1970s as the primary health care providers in the Monroe area. In the late 1970s, however, reimbursement cutbacks, increased costs, capital investment needs in facilities and equipment, and leadership transition caused each organization to focus on its individual concerns. As the Hospital and Clinic began to deal with internal issues, service competition emerged; eventually, communication and joint planning between the two organizations were diminished.

Continued financial concerns, leadership turnover, and uncertainty about the future health care environment led both organizations to conclude that some form of consolidation was needed. The result was a formal affiliation that has strengthened both the Hospital and the Clinic.

☐ Background

Monroe, Wisconsin, is a rural area located in the southern part of the state—south of Madison and just north of the Illinois border (northwest of Rockford, Illinois). With a population of approximately 10,000, the town has a strong agricultural base with most of its dairy products devoted to cheese production. Monroe has a stable, diversified industrial base and exceptionally low unemployment, with a small Medicaid and indigent population.

In the early 1990s, managed care products represented less than 10 percent of the health insurance products offered to the population of Monroe. There were virtually no capitated insurance programs in the community.

Hospital

The 174-bed St. Clare Hospital is sponsored by the Congregation of the Sisters of St. Agnes. The nearest competitor hospital is located in Freeport, Illinois, approximately 26 miles south of St. Clare Hospital. Monroe's medical community has a patient draw area of a 100-mile radius.

Clinic

The Clinic experienced rapid growth during its first 30 years and grew into a 50-plus multispecialty physician group. Clinic physicians, along with the anesthesiology, radiology, and orthopedic groups, comprise the Hospital's active medical staff. The Clinic has a main office in Monroe, with 10 branch locations throughout the area.

A consumer study identified three reasons why the Hospital and Clinic have a strong patient preference rating in a large market geographic area. First, a number of patients enjoy "one-stop" delivery, having their health care needs met in one trip. For example, they can visit their primary care physician, have diagnostic studies done, consult a specialist, and receive a diagnostic summary from their primary care physician—all in one day. Second, patients are not treated by interns and residents, as is the case in the suburban centers. Third, the Hospital and the Clinic are known for their high level of quality throughout the region.

Hospital–Clinic Relations

Despite the fact that Clinic physicians comprise more than 90 percent of the Hospital's medical staff, by the early 1980s relations between Hospital and Clinic had become strained. The Clinic's founders, who had worked with the Hospital over the years to ensure the growth of both organizations, were retiring. As leadership shifted to the next generation of physicians, the Clinic's desire to work more closely with the Hospital continued, despite the fact that physicians began more openly to articulate goal conflicts between the two organizations.

Because of concern over decreasing reimbursement, Clinic physicians were reluctant to invest in the future growth and value of the Clinic. Senior physicians nearing retirement feared the prospect of carrying the liability of capital investment in the Clinic into their final years of practice. Their interest was in maintaining maximum value for their buyout from Clinic ownership. This period saw all Clinic investment focused on areas with near-term return on investment, such as expanded ancillary services.

Pressure from senior physicians to maximize Clinic revenues and income distribution to physician owners was driven by a growing concern over reduced reimbursement levels by third-party payers and government programs. For example, the Clinic did not participate in the Medicare program.

In the mid-1970s, the Clinic hired a consultant to assist in developing systems, policies, and services to maximize income. On the advice of the consultant, the Clinic developed outpatient services (diagnostic imaging, laboratory services, physical therapy, and pharmacy services) in competition with existing Hospital services.

At the same time, the Hospital was addressing its own internal issues. The introduction of Medicare DRG reimbursement greatly reduced Hospital income, and to offset this reduction in revenues, management focused on cost reduction and expansion of outpatient services. The Hospital did not have a strategic planning process in place and, given the Clinic's internal focus, did not devote management effort to medical staff relations. Hospital administrators, of course, were unhappy about the Clinic's development of competing services.

In the midst of this turmoil, the Hospital board expressed a growing concern over the Hospital's ability to carry out its mission to provide services to the medically indigent in its service area.

The board hired a new Hospital president in 1982. One of his primary charges was to improve hospital–medical staff relations and to develop a joint strategic plan with the Clinic.

Early Collaborative Efforts

A strategic planning process was begun in 1983 with the Hospital board and administration and the physician leadership of the Monroe Clinic. Despite agreement that joint efforts were needed, after several months' discussion the only mutual agenda arrived at was joint marketing to Monroe's medical community through advertising and direct mail; provision of patient and physician education programs; recruitment of new physicians to meet community need and replace retiring physicians; and continued joint planning activities.

The Monroe Regional Medical Center was established in 1984 as a joint not-for-profit company devoted to promoting Monroe's medical community in the service area and surrounding communities. This effort was successful in developing marketing materials and conducting patient education programs, among other activities. As a result of these activities, out-migration of inpatient admissions was reduced. Funding for this effort was minimal and was split 60/40 between the Hospital and Clinic respectively.

In late 1986, a formal strategic plan, approved by the Hospital and the Monroe Clinic, outlined the need for the two organizations to continue working together. This decision led to creation of the Monroe Health Services Management Organization (MHSMO). A Hospital–Clinic partnership designed to formally address joint issues such as physician recruitment and the establishment of branch Clinic offices, MHSMO had no significant start-up costs.

Both of these early collaborative efforts were incorporated as separate entities from the Hospital and the Clinic. In both instances, the organizations leased employees from one or both of the constituents and were governed by a board made up of representatives from the Hospital and the Clinic. (See figure 12-1.)

Over the next several years, Monroe Clinic had difficulty supporting decisions reached by these jointly sponsored organizations. Because physicians assigned as Clinic representatives to the MHSMO were not board members, they had little real authority. Consequently, they had little success getting Clinic approval of MHSMO actions. Trust between the Hospital and Clinic fell to an all-time low.

Two strategic plans were developed over the next six years, but it was difficult to achieve consensus from the Clinic and the Hospital. The Clinic resisted the Hospital's pressure to make the ancillary services a joint venture. After a long tenure, the Clinic administrator retired in the late 1980s, leaving Clinic leadership in transition.

Clinic Leadership Change

The president and vice-president of the Clinic, both in their 30s, were elected in 1989. Their mandate was to find a way to expand Clinic services and update facilities without splitting the Clinic along lines of financial interests of individual physicians. Historically there had been no accumulation of financial reserves for long-term planning and investment. Older physicians resisted current investment that would benefit the younger physicians over time but have a negative impact on current Clinic income. However, given the new political power of the younger physicians, the majority of physicians supported modernization of facilities and recruitment of new physicians.

Figure 12-1. Organizational Structure Showing Early Attempts at Integration

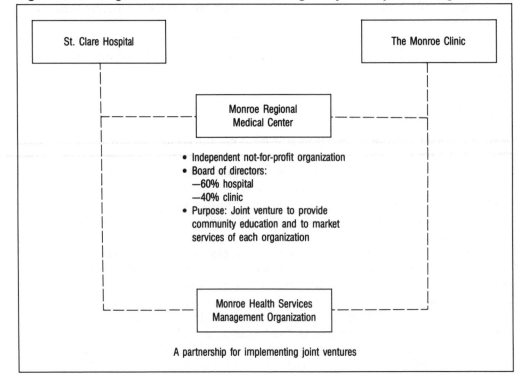

☐ Motivations to Collaborate

The new Clinic leadership recognized the need for strategic planning and capital investment if the group was to survive. A seminar on hospital–physician joint ventures sharpened their awareness of the benefits of joint efforts. The leaders of both organizations followed up by studying hospital–physician affiliations in other communities.

In response to the Clinic's needs for capital to update and expand its facilities, the Hospital offered to build a medical building on its campus to house the Clinic—but with the stipulation that ancillary services would be consolidated with the Hospital. Amid strong reaction to this proposal, including several physicians leaving the Clinic, the Clinic still had financial concerns. Each organization continued to address its needs and goals for the future, eventually recognizing that mutual benefits could be gained from collaboration.

Clinic Motivations

The Clinic's three orthopedic surgeons, concerned over the prospect of losing revenues from ancillary services through joint venture with the Hospital in conjunction with a new hospital-owned facility, left the Clinic. Because they were the highest revenue producers in the group, other physicians saw their departure as a threat to the Clinic's financial outlook.

In late 1989, an additional exodus from the group occurred when the three-physician cardiology department dissolved. One physician retired, one joined a pharmaceutical company to pursue his research interest, and the third left under the stress of trying single-handedly to maintain the caseload with few prospects for recruitment of a new cardiologist. The financial impact from the loss of these physicians was significant. The Hospital and Clinic cooperated to contract with a group of out-of-town cardiologists to provide inpatient and outpatient services until new cardiologists could be recruited.

Despite increasing receptiveness to joint efforts with the Hospital, its offer to create an on-campus Clinic office building and to joint venture ancillary services was rejected. Instead, the physicians elected to pursue development of a new building on their own. Their decision was met with resistance by a minority of physicians concerned over the Clinic's shrinking revenues, physician departures, and the need for expansion to meet patient and payer demands.

In planning for the new building, the group found it difficult to reach consensus on design and space assignment. Designs were changed repeatedly and costs rose as each physician sought the best facilities for his or her individual practice.

By spring 1991, Clinic leaders recognized that they could not build and expand on their own. At the same time, the presidency of the group was assumed by a young, well-respected rheumatologist whose inheritance was a group nervous about the future and dissatisfied with past actions of the Clinic.

Concern over the departure of high-revenue producers in the group was magnified by anxiety over new building costs, recruitment of replacements for the retiring physicians, and increasing operating expenses. These financial crises reflected the lack of appropriate planning that had characterized Clinic operations over the past years. The new president recognized the group's critical need for new facilities and expansion. He devoted his energies to maintaining consensus among the physicians on these needs *and* seeking solutions that would not cause the group insurmountable financial hardships.

Hospital Motivations

The Hospital sought the stability of the large group practice that constituted the majority of its medical staff and as early as 1983 had committed to continued joint planning with the medical staff to deal with the changing health care environment. The Hospital also was dealing with reduced revenues from ancillary services as a result of the duplication of services created by the Clinic's recent addition and expansion of ancillary departments.

Recruiting physicians to replace retiring physicians and meeting the demands of the community it served were two of the organization's priorities. Also, the requirements for geographic coverage by primary care providers under managed care contracts made the Clinic's survival essential for successful contracting. Erosion of the group could reduce the Hospital's branch Clinic network, compromise the Hospital's physician recruitment effort, and ultimately limit its ability to contract with managed care products.

☐ Planning Process

Clinic and Hospital leaders began educating the physicians as to potential benefits of a formal affiliation. With the aid of outside speakers, Hospital administrators facilitated discussions with the Clinic physicians as to the Clinic's goals for the future and what role the Hospital could play in achieving these goals. This process was supported by the new leadership at the Clinic and their commitment to advancing Clinic–Hospital relations.

Awareness and Issues Identification

Hospital administrators proposed a formal affiliation planning process, which began with discussions of the historical and future relationship between the two organizations. Both agreed to forging a partnership, with each taking responsibility in its areas of proven expertise. (See figure 12-2.)

The Hospital provided data to convince physicians of the benefits of an affiliation. Encouraged by their visits to other integrated organizations, as well as by the educational efforts of the Hospital, Clinic leaders became aware of the potential benefits of a Hospital–physician affiliation and spread the word to other Clinic physicians. Emphasis was placed on how a collaboration would help physician practices meet current and future financial and operational needs while ensuring their survival in a changing health care climate.

In regard to specific issues, both organizations acknowledged that hospitals and physician practices traditionally had different goals and missions, financial strategies, billing systems, and management structures. The planning group identified the critical needs to be addressed in a collaboration; for example, ability to share risk under capitated reimbursement and managed care contracting, and cost-effective resource utilization in providing care to the community. The negative financial impact of competing services was identified, as was the Clinic's need for capital to upgrade facilities. Pending retirements and physician departures, based on financial or personal issues, threatened the ability of both organizations to provide the level of care they had offered in the past and created a critical need for successful physician recruitment. Finally, the planning group addressed its need to maintain the quality of medical services provided to the community, as well as to expand the group's patient draw area.

Figure 12-2. Affiliated Relationship Planning: Areas of Responsibility

Hospital	Clinic	Joint Effort
• Inpatient services—management and operations • Clinic services—management and operations • Financial planning and management	• Medical issues—inpatient and outpatient • Physician recruitment • Physician compensation	• Strategic planning • Marketing • Managed care contracting • Addition of services

Issues Resolution

During the planning process, both organizations recognized their differences in terms of culture, values, management styles, and decision-making processes. Timetables were set and meetings scheduled to address specific issues identified by the planning group and to arrive at mutually acceptable strategies for resolution. For example, sterilizations were performed in the Clinic because the Catholic mission prohibited performance of these procedures in the Hospital. Upon reaching a consensus on goals of the affiliated organization, a compromise was reached. The Monroe Medical Foundation for Education and Research, a structure set up by the Clinic for educational and research support, would be maintained as a separate entity in a separate facility. Sterilization procedures would be scheduled and billed through the foundation, and receipts from these activities would go to the foundation.

Awareness development led to identification of specific issues to be resolved in creating a Hospital–Clinic affiliation. (See figure 12-3.) The consensus, however, was that consultants and attorneys would not be brought into the process until the Clinic and Hospital had reached agreement on "conceptual resolution" of issues and it was time to address the details. In addition, it was agreed that issues having the most potential for easy resolution would be addressed first.

Key Benefits of Consolidation

In discussing key benefits the Hospital and Clinic would gain through an affiliation, both organizations agreed that improved quality of care to the community at a reduced cost could be accomplished with reduction of overhead cost. This would be achieved through use of consolidated resources and services. With reduction in capital costs, physician recruitment and service expansion could be facilitated.

Planning Results

Ultimately, the Hospital's decision to purchase Clinic assets and employ the physicians evolved from this process of issues resolution and benefits identification. Because of the physicians' desire to retain autonomy in their practice operations, initial investigations centered on Hospital ownership of assets only, with the Clinic retaining the practice and leasing assets and management services from the Hospital. This structure would assure physicians of having control over practice policies, physician income distribution, recruitment, and other areas. The Clinic would retain its board, which would negotiate the lease with the Hospital.

Under the planning group's scrutiny of the Clinic's financial situation both in terms of reduced revenues and investment required for facilities and equipment, this structure presented more legal and regulatory concerns. The Hospital could not subsidize the lease or costs for management services to a private physician group without jeopardizing the

Figure 12-3. Issues to Be Resolved prior to Affiliation

- Physician's role in policy direction and operations of an affiliated organization
  —Physician representation and influence on boards, committees, and other decision-making bodies
  —Physicians in top-level management
- Financing construction of a new clinic facility
- Consolidation of ancillary services
- Resolution of issues related to the religious affiliation of the Hospital (sterilization procedures)
- Physician compensation under the affiliation
- Maintenance of the integrity of the physician group
- Maintenance of the Clinic's identification

Hospital's tax-exempt status through exposure under the private inurement regulations. Any support to the physician group was also subject to scrutiny under Medicare fraud and abuse regulations.

The legal and structural requirements of maintaining the Clinic as a separate entity not only would delay consolidation but also might hamper the organizations' achievement of the agreed-on goals of affiliation. Therefore the decision was made that the Hospital would employ the physicians. Discussions then moved to finalize the design of the new organization, the purchase price for the Clinic assets, physician compensation under the new organization, and available alternatives to the Hospital and Clinic should the plans for merger be rejected.

Presentation of Plan

Clinic leaders presented the affiliation plan to the Clinic's shareholders. A major component of this presentation was the review of year-end financial information and options for the organization's future. The following options were presented to the group:

- Maintain status quo (no building program)
- Construct a new building and assume the associated cost within the Clinic
- Seek buyout or affiliation with other physician groups
- Consolidate with St. Clare Hospital

The presentation and discussion clearly demonstrated the financial problems that confronted the physicians failing access to capital through an affiliation, thus eliminating the first two options. The physicians expressed concern about potential loss of operational autonomy for the Clinic if affiliated with a partner from outside the local community, as described in the third option. Finally, consolidation with the Hospital, the last option, was presented in detail, along with a discussion of trends in mergers and affiliations between hospitals and group practices. A consolidation plan was presented and accepted in principle by the group.

Prior to the shareholders' meeting, physician leaders met with each physician in the group one-on-one to discuss the possibilities of integration, address each physician's concerns, and build consensus. Thus, at the meeting, the physicians unanimously voted to sign a letter of intent to consolidate with the Hospital. (See figure 12-4.)

☐ Negotiations

The negotiations team focused on resolving conceptual issues identified in the planning process rather than dealing with specific line-item issues, which were left for attorneys and accountants to work out. Specific tasks included assessing practice value, integrating employees into the new structure, consolidating ancillary services, designing a physician compensation package, and determining financing needs.

Practice Valuation

Purchase of the practice involved assets only. These included cash; building, equipment, and land; prepaid insurance; inventory; and net accounts receivable.

External resources were used to develop a valuation basis and approach, but the ultimate value was agreed to internally by the Hospital and Clinic. If the asset values changed by a preestablished amount by the closing date, it was agreed that the final purchase price would reflect the asset value at time of closing.

A key success factor in the valuation process was the negotiating team's constant focus on the *total purchase price*. That is, each item was not negotiated individually but

Figure 12-4. Components of the Letter of Intent

Binding Provisions

- Make best efforts to reach final agreement
- Define issues of governance and management prior to formalizing a binding agreement
- Focus on conceptual issues during negotiation, with details to be worked out during implementation
- Exchange all information with commitment to confidentiality
- Utilize legal and financial counsel to address details as agreement on the basic issues are reached
- Maintain exclusivity in dealings between the parties
- Maintain ordinary course of business during negotiations

Nonbinding Provisions

- Proceed toward consolidation
- Develop a statement of objectives and outline of proposed organizational structures
- Maintain the integrity of the physician group
- Investigate facility relocation
- Address goals and objectives of physician compensation
- Pursue appropriate due diligence
- Address Catholic sponsorship issues
- Define assets purchase price
- Agree to operation of ancillaries after affiliation
- Define employment status of Clinic employees
- Address tax-exempt issues
- Pursue a one-year time frame for achieving consolidation
- Investigate existing contractual obligations
- Address operational issues of concern to both parties

assigned a fair price, with the overall price for the entire enterprise kept in mind. Both parties were aware of private inurement issues in the purchase of the for-profit Clinic by the not-for-profit Hospital.

The biggest asset item was accounts receivable; other assets were valued at fair market value and agreed to easily. The Clinic had over $6 million of accounts receivable on the books, with an allowance of $1 million for uncollectibles. The Hospital believed the allowance for uncollectibles was inadequate, which was confirmed through outside consultants. Final agreement on the value of accounts receivable was $5 million. No breakdown of accounts receivable was made based on age; the value was determined on the entire balance.

No payment was made for practice goodwill. Issues of fraud and abuse and private inurement, the Clinic's financial outlook without benefit of affiliation, and the physicians' concern with survival of the group all compelled acceptance of this arrangement. If the Clinic dissolved, the physicians would be faced with prohibitive costs for restarting their practices independently.

Employee Integration

In addressing differences in salaries, benefits, and personnel policies between the two settings, it was agreed that the Hospital would absorb the Clinic employees, although job requirements, responsibility, and hours for similar positions differed. The Hospital agreed to undertake a post-purchase job measurement and evaluation process to establish compensation after fair assessment of each job.

The employee benefits package did cause concern for Clinic employees, whose pension benefit was approximately 10 percent of salary. The Hospital plans worked out to approximately 8.5 percent of employee salary, but the Hospital also provided dental coverage (which the Clinic had not) and more vacation time. Adjusting to being Hospital employees has not been without problems for former Clinic employees. Personnel policies and procedures, ranging from disciplinary action to job evaluation, have changed. The Clinic employees have also been concerned about their ongoing job security.

Hospital employees also found many of the changes difficult. The consolidation has resulted in eliminating duplication of services and functions, with corresponding staffing adjustments that raise fears among Hospital employees about elimination of positions, reduced working hours, and other security concerns.

To help ease transition anxiety, each employee of both organizations was given the book *How to Survive a Merger.*[1] Meetings were held to promote a common philosophy in the new organization and to help employees understand that it could take several years to reach true integration of the staffs.

Ancillary Services

Physicians agreed that the cost of maintaining duplicate ancillary services was prohibitive. Therefore, these services are being consolidated, with the new Clinic facility creating a common campus with the Hospital. To accommodate the increased volume in ancillary services, $7.5 million was spent on Hospital renovation.

Physician Compensation

With an agreement in principle that physicians should be paid a fair salary based on work performed as compared with peers, an outside consultant was brought in to help design a compensation package. The Medical Group Management Association (MGMA) annual physician productivity and income survey was used as a basis for comparison.

Clinic physician net revenue (exclusive of ancillary services) was monitored for individual physicians. Each salary would be determined by applying the specialty-specific overhead factor (established by MGMA surveys of group practice physicians) to each physician's net revenue. This method met the criterion of reasonable compensation for services rendered that is required of tax-exempt organizations. "Market pay for market work" continues to be the philosophy behind physician compensation.

Financing

The Hospital determined that approximately $29.5 million would be required to accomplish this merger. Funds were allocated as follows:

- Purchase of Monroe Clinic assets—$9.5 million
- Construction of a new medical office building—$12.5 million
- Hospital renovations—$7.5 million

After consulting a number of experts on the best approach for financing this consolidation, the Hospital determined that a rated bond issue with tax-exempt financing would be best. The issuing authority would be a Wisconsin Health and Educational Facility Authority, and the revenue bonds would be a public issue. Experts consulted for development of the issue included financial advisers, underwriters, bond rating agencies, bond trustees, issuing authority counsel, Hospital counsel, and a feasibility study consultant.

In May 1992 the negotiations were completed and agreements signed. The planning and negotiation processes that led to consolidation occurred over a 10-year period, beginning with the initial commitment in the early 1980s. The time line for the joint process is shown in figure 12-5.

☐ Implementation

Throughout the planning and negotiating efforts, meetings were held constantly with physicians, individually and in groups. These meetings continued throughout the

Figure 12-5. Affiliation Time Line

1983	Joint strategic planning process began between Clinic and Hospital
1983	Formation of Monroe Health Services Management Organization (MHSMO)—partnership to implement joint market strategies
1983	Formation of Monroe Regional Medical Center (MRMC), which is a not-for-profit organization. A joint effort for marketing and community education began
1988	Election of new Clinic leadership
1988	Offer by Hospital to build a new Clinic building on Hospital campus
1990	Clinic announces plans to remodel and expand its office building on existing site
Spring 1991	Hospital board of directors meets informally with Clinic leadership to discuss integration
Summer 1991	Informal visits of Hospital and Clinic leadership to integrated health facilities
Fall 1991	Informal discussions begin concerning integration
Mid-November 1991	Formal presentation of options to Monroe Clinic shareholders
Late November 1991	Letter of intent to integrate Hospital and Clinic unanimously approved
April 17, 1992	Bonds are approved and sold
May 4, 1992	Consolidation formally occurs with assets of Clinic purchased by Hospital
November 1993	New Clinic facility opens on Hospital campus and organization changes its name to The Monroe Clinic

implementation process but were expanded to other levels of involvement: group meetings with supervisors and managers from both organizations; employee meetings with the Hospital and Clinic presidents; and meetings between Hospital–Clinic representatives and community leaders and other groups in the service area. All communication efforts—including news conferences and news releases—served to announce the Hospital–Clinic affiliation and address physician and employee concerns (fear of the unknown, power struggles, mistrust, job security, and so forth).

A joint letter was developed for Hospital and Clinic employees. The letter described how the integration of the Hospital and Clinic would benefit employees and the community as well as how integration would mutually benefit the Hospital and Clinic in achieving their respective missions. To facilitate the transition the Hospital hired a Clinic administrator, an individual with extensive medical group practice management experience who quickly gained the physicians' confidence. A consultant also was engaged to assist with managing the emotional aspects of integration, particularly with respect to adjustment to different missions and management approaches and to environmental change.

The implementation process fostered a sense of unity and a positive outlook for the future. Physicians, bolstered by the strength of consolidation, prepared to address strategic planning for their group practice. There was a sense of empowerment, ownership, and enthusiasm for the new organization and its potential growth and commitment to enhanced patient services.

☐ Future Outlook

As indicated, the impact of the merger on Clinic operations during the first year has been in terms of positive, measurable outcomes. Several issues, however, have been identified that affect future success:

- *Physician compensation:* The new compensation formula has resulted in physician salaries being higher than when the Clinic was a freestanding facility. This is due primarily to the high overhead the Clinic experienced prior to the merger. Expected operational savings realized from consolidation that will reduce operating expenses are budgeted to offset this increase. Future adjustments in compensation structures are anticipated as managed care contracting increases.
- *Physician benefits:* The commitment to provide stability and security for physicians throughout the integration remains intact, with benefits continuing at previously established levels.
- *Personnel issues:* A compensation assessment has been initiated to determine appropriate salary and benefits for employees. This issue continues to create apprehension among employees, and efforts to maintain open communication continue.
- *Management functions:* As the integrated organization begins to develop budgets and strategic plans and to follow through on decisions, understanding and overcoming differences continues to challenge the organization.
- *Managed care:* A partnership with an insurance company has been established to provide regional employers with various health insurance products. The insurance company was selected following response to a request for proposal subsequent to the Hospital's purchase of the Clinic. In the first few months, 1,500 employees were enrolled. Current premiums and reimbursement are based on a fee schedule, but negotiations are under way to develop capitated products. The insurance company provides claims processing services and utilization data. The current outlook is good.
- *Organization name:* Following completion of the new facility, the organization changed its name to The Monroe Clinic. This name change reflects the commitment of both the Hospital and the Clinic to unifying the new organization to provide high-quality, cost-effective health care to its patients.
- *Consolidation goals:* The organization is moving quickly to combine services, staffing, and resources by relocating the Clinic to the Hospital campus. This cost-saving move, the insurance company partnership, and a Hospital and physician commitment to control costs all are designed to position the Monroe Clinic as an accountable health plan as defined in the Clinton administration health care reform proposals.

Reference

1. Pritchett, P. *How to Survive a Merger.* Dallas: Pritchett Publishing, 1987.

Chapter 13
Summary of Case Study Findings

☐ Introduction

The U.S. health care delivery system is undergoing a period of dramatic changes influenced by political, social, and economic factors. Providers must develop new organizational structures if they are to continue providing the quality of care that meets their standard and survive in a new economic environment.

Many hospitals and physicians are pursuing a hospital–group practice affiliation as a key component in addressing these changes. The diverse elements of an affiliation and its planning, development, negotiation, and implementation processes, as shown in this book—particularly the case studies—reflect the complexity of issues that surround this joint effort.

There is no set formula for success. Rather, the circumstances of each hospital and physician group must guide the collective process to identify an appropriate affiliation structure. The case studies further demonstrate that affiliations are evolutionary by nature, requiring strong leadership and flexibility to adopt to the changing health care environment.

Also as demonstrated throughout this book, each case is unique in terms of geographic location and service area, facility size, patient population, and the like. Even so, five factors are common to each setting and critically influence the outcome of joint efforts:

1. Local health care environment
2. Hospital and physician goals and objectives
3. The relationship between hospital and physicians
4. The planning and negotiation atmosphere
5. The availability of strong leaders, capable managers, and flexible systems

This chapter will present these factors (and their "subfactors") with a view of bringing together findings from the seven case studies. The conclusions drawn can be applied as a generic guide for an entity considering affiliation as an option. None of these conclusions, however, is intended to substitute for experienced legal counsel and financial advisers.

☐ Environment

To create a hospital–group practice affiliation, planners must understand not only the larger health care picture but also the local environment in which the hospitals and physicians provide care. Community standards and health care needs, level of competition among providers, number of existing physician group practices, and the penetration of capitated reimbursement into the marketplace are key influencers on a hospital–group practice affiliation.

Community Need

An identified need for additional physicians in the community will affect the structure and physician makeup of a hospital-affiliated group practice. For example, hospitals can establish new group practices staffed by newly recruited physicians. Alternatively, in an environment where physician supply is adequate to meet community demand, a hospital may integrate existing practices—those affiliated with its medical staff and those loyal to competitor hospitals. Failure to identify a community need for additional providers can lead to slow patient volume and stunted revenue growth in a new practice. On the other hand, a community needs assessment can help determine which type of physicians (primary care or specialist) to recruit into the community, how many are needed, and appropriate locations for group practice sites. Community need can be influenced by the out-migration of patients or by the pending retirement of existing physicians. Community needs assessment also serves to document physician recruitment needs and practice start-up support provided to a new physician by a hospital relative to private inurement and Medicare fraud and abuse issues.

Competition

Competition for patient admissions or managed care contracts often is a catalyst for hospitals to take steps to secure loyalty among their medical staff. The development of a hospital-affiliated group practice is a good vehicle toward this end and can provide access to the hospital's services through expanded geographic accessibility to a larger population.

With emphasis on the gatekeeper role of primary care in the changing health care delivery system, hospitals are aggressively seeking affiliations with primary care providers. Competition among specialists for referrals from primary care physicians can lead to specialists' support for hospital activities directed toward expansion of a loyal primary care base through a primary care group practice.

In today's environment, hospitals must be aware that competition will come from new sources as integrated providers develop partnerships with managed care products that can be marketed to expanded geographic areas. Tertiary care hospitals, which traditionally relied on referrals from outlying community hospitals, will seek to develop a direct primary care presence in an extended service area. This activity can create competition for smaller hospitals in these outlying areas. A hospital-affiliated group practice can provide a community hospital a defense against this expanding competition.

Existing Group Practices

Hospital affiliations with existing group practices create a set of circumstances different from those inherent in newly established group practices, which integrate existing physicians or recruit new physicians. Major differences fall into categories as described in the following subsections.

Strategic Planning
Group practices often devote more time to addressing long-term practice strategies than do solo practitioners, who focus on more tactical, short-term needs. Physicians in a group

practice recognize more readily the long-term goals and objectives in working with the hospital and, therefore, recognize the benefit an affiliated structure brings to their practice.

Negotiations

Negotiations for hospital affiliation with an existing group may require more time and energy than that demanded for new group negotiations. Existing solo practitioners, seeking resolution to tactical needs, can quickly identify the benefits of joining a newly affiliated hospital group practice. Candidates being recruited to the community for a group practice are concerned primarily with compensation, work hours, practice environment, and such basic issues. Conversely, an existing group practice focuses negotiations on the longer-term issues of control and direction of the group after affiliation; this is because members have built up experiential equity in group practice operations. These issues require more negotiation time to reach an agreement on structure, ownership, and control.

Initial capital costs for the purchase of an existing group practice can be higher than costs of gradually developing a group through the integration of existing practices or recruitment of new physicians. The hospital must deal with a larger initial capital investment in negotiating the deal.

Physician Leadership

An existing group practice will have an already-established structure of physician leaders, which can move along the implementation process (although, as mentioned, it can add to negotiation time). However, the hospital must ensure that the physician leaders understand the goals and objectives of the affiliation and that they have the support of their practice constituents. A group practice facing financial crisis through decreasing patient volumes or revenues may also be experiencing support shortage or instability with its leadership.

Group Practice Management and Operating Systems

Implementation of an affiliated group practice developed from multiple existing practices or the recruitment of new physicians can be complicated by the absence of group practice management experience. This deficit can contribute to failure to implement the systems required for efficient operations. This problem should not exist in an affiliation with an existing group, where management resources and systems are already in place. However, the hospital should investigate the existing operations to determine their effectiveness, efficiency, and compatibility and to identify any resources that may be needed to ensure a smooth transition.

Managed Care Penetration

As the reimbursement rules for services rendered by physicians change under managed care insurance products, physicians recognize the need to modify their practice operations in order to survive economically. Transition from fee-for-service to capitated reimbursement mandates these changes. A group practice can provide a vehicle for physicians to incorporate these changes into their practice patterns. Use of physician extenders, consolidation of services, and physician commitment to utilization control can be implemented more effectively in a group practice environment. Physicians are reluctant to change traditional practice patterns so long as 60 percent or more of their revenue comes through traditional fee-for-service reimbursement. This influences their willingness to accept the long-term strategies identified by a hospital, including risk sharing, contracting, resource consolidation, and acceptance of treatment protocols. The implementation of changes through a hospital-affiliated group practice can be supported through the strategic planning process as well as financial support for needed resources, but change is still slower where there is less capitated reimbursement and therefore less direct financial motivation for physicians.

The willingness of existing solo practitioners to join a hospital-affiliated group practice is also enhanced by a high level of penetration by capitated reimbursement. The need to have a larger population over which to spread risk through expanded geographic accessibility motivates the physicians to seek a group practice environment. The need to utilize resources effectively and reduce the cost of care delivery further motivates physicians to form groups in an environment with significant capitated reimbursement.

□ Goals and Objectives

Hospital-affiliated group practices may achieve a variety of goals and objectives for the hospital and physicians. In some cases, immediate issues are addressed, for example, short-term goals such as funding for capital to upgrade or expand practice facilities or the creation of a practice structure that will appeal to physician candidates being recruited to the community. Longer-term strategic goals may also be addressed through an affiliation, for example, development of an integrated delivery system to meet the challenges of a changing health care environment or consolidation of ancillary services to reduce the cost of health care to a patient population.

The case studies are evidence that a hospital-affiliated group practice becomes a key element in pursuing the long-term strategic goals of the hospital and its medical staff, whatever the original motivations might have been. Thus, the hospital and physicians must recognize the long-term impact an affiliated group practice will have on the current structures for delivery of care and its potential to make a positive impact on health care delivery.

Hospital Motivations

Traditionally, hospitals more than physician practices have developed long-range strategic plans. This is because hospitals are established with the mission to serve the community's health care needs in perpetuity. Unlike physician practices, a hospital's existence does not revolve around an individual, who must sell or otherwise transfer the practice to another physician for it to survive. Compensation of hospital leaders is not directly contingent on their organizations' bottom line, therefore affording them a longer-term perspective from which to develop strategic plans.

This does not mean that hospitals may not be motivated by short-term strategies. Protecting their medical staff and referral base to retain admissions, expanding ambulatory services, or responding to immediate competition for managed care contracts all represent potential short-term motivations.

In most cases, however, hospitals recognize the *strategic importance* of affiliation to the long-term success of both the hospital and physician practices. This understanding should be incorporated into the planning and negotiation focus so as to avoid internal conflict down the road. Affiliated structures established to meet only short-term needs often require major changes as the group practice becomes more significantly integrated into the hospital's operations and budget.

The hospital must balance the resources committed to developing an affiliated group practice against providing support to medical staff members who do not participate in the group practice. Ensuring that *all* medical staff understand the strategic importance of the affiliation will help alleviate concerns over the hospital's focus. In most cases, the physician participants—usually primary care physicians only—represent a small part of the entire staff.

Hospitals and physicians often underestimate the financial commitment required to develop an affiliated group practice. Table 13-1 reflects the first-year investment per full-time physician for five of the case studies in this book. Whether purchasing existing practices or starting new ones, hospital leaders must justify the substantial financial

Table 13-1. First-Year Investment per Full-Time Physician

Institution	Number of Physicians	First-Year Investment	First-Year Investment per Full-Time Physician
Good Samaritan San Jose, CA	18	$ 9,000,000[a]	$500,000
Millard Fillmore Buffalo, NY	1	$ 552,425[b]	$550,000
Mercy Hospital Pittsburgh, PA	3	$ 680,000[c]	$226,000
St. Luke's Saginaw, MI	1	$ 130,200[b]	$130,000
Monroe Clinic Monroe, WI	41	$29,500,000[d]	$720,000

[a]Includes first-year payment for group practice purchase and budgeted operating losses.
[b]Includes first-year operating results including renovations and equipping of practice site and practice losses.
[c]Includes first-year budget for facility improvement, equipment and furnishings, start-up costs (projected operating losses).
[d]Includes first-year budget for purchase of group practice, building new facility, hospital renovations, and operating losses.

commitment to their boards on the basis of the long-term strategic importance of the endeavor. Therefore, a realistic business plan must balance the proposed investment against the impact an affiliated group will have on the hospital's overall operations and revenues.

Strategic implications also apply to development of support services. Traditionally, hospital managers and supervisors are trained to treat all physicians equally and to avoid fanning the flames of conflict and dissent that can be sparked by favoritism. Because of the high patient volume, group practices rely on flexibility and responsiveness from all support departments—from maintenance to purchasing, personnel, and billing. Therefore, appreciation of the strategic importance of the affiliated group practice must be disseminated organizationwide.

Physician Motivations

As mentioned, small groups or solo practitioners tend to focus on short-term needs—concerns over patient volume, access to capital, financial security, and reduction of managerial burdens. However, risk sharing and managed care penetration (as discussed in a preceding section) can spur practitioners to long-term planning.

Aside from retention of autonomy, physicians must be comfortable with appointment scheduling, resource availability (ancillary staffing, examination rooms and equipment, medical records, and so forth), and other practice operations. Under pressure to modify their practice patterns so as to address patients' long-term medical needs versus episodic care, group practitioners must be assured a reasonable level of compensation. A hospital affiliation can provide a vehicle to support physicians during practice transition, necessary adjustments to their practice patterns, and realignment of practice operations.

☐ Relationship between Hospitals and Physicians

Before deciding to join a group practice, physicians must first trust that the goals and objectives of the group are compatible with their personal standards of care delivery and business operations. Physicians rely on making independent judgments on their patients'

211

behalf, an orientation reinforced particularly for solo practitioners, who in effect have become small business entrepreneurs. Therefore physicians, personally vested in their practices, measure their personal and practice success against their standing in the community.

These concerns are compounded when a hospital enters the picture as a potential partner, because the physician reputation is now tied to that of the hospital as well as to others in the group. Therefore, a key building block in a hospital–group practice affiliation is a relationship of mutual respect and trust between the hospital leaders and the physicians. They must agree that their goals, objectives, strategies, and philosophies are compatible.

This relationship is shaped by four elements. The first is the historical context of the hospital–physician relationship; the second is the experience of having arrived at mutual goals; the third is the personal involvement of top leaders during planning and negotiations; and the fourth is the style of governance and level of control agreed to for the affiliated practice.

Historical Relationship

The traditional relationship between hospitals and their medical staff has created more conflict than consensus. Physicians, concerned primarily with making sick patients better, perceive that *how* care is delivered is the physician's responsibility. Hospital managers, concerned primarily with costs and utilization efficiencies, perceive that physicians' autonomy may conflict with administrative priorities. This conflict may carry over to ownership and control of ancillary services. For example, physicians seeking to enhance service to their patients and practice revenues have developed sophisticated outpatient ambulatory services in their offices—outside the hospital. At the same time, the hospital seeks to utilize those resources acquired for the delivery of *inpatient* care in providing *outpatient* ancillary services.

Historically at cross-purposes, hospital managers may react with skepticism to physician requests for additional in-hospital equipment or services on behalf of their patients. At the same time, physicians may perceive the hospital's focus on long-term planning and retained earnings to fund future needs as an inappropriate response to the immediate demands of their patients.

Physicians are privy to internal hospital operations through participation on medical staff committees and planning committees and as officers and board representatives. Given their entrepreneurial orientation, physicians characterize hospitals as bureaucratic organizations that are nonresponsive to the needs of their customers (that is, the physicians and patients). Hospital managers, however, do not have comparable exposure to a physician's practice and consequently have little direct knowledge of the demands of high patient volume and personal relationships between physician and patients in the practice. Until this "exposure gap" is bridged, understanding one another's needs and priorities will continue to challenge hospitals and physicians in efforts to create compatible goals and structures for a hospital-affiliated group practice.

Historical successes in working with physicians in developing new programs, providing services to medical practices, or contracting with insurance companies can enhance the relationship. Failures in past efforts can lead to distrust on both sides in planning future affiliations.

The point here is that the historical relationship between a hospital and the physicians who will participate in the affiliated group practice must be addressed. A poor relationship must be repaired before planning begins. Furthermore, poor hospital–medical staff relations can negatively affect hospital-developed group practices staffed by new physician recruits. This problem can surface with failure to attract candidates following site visits and high turnover among new recruits.

Mutual Goals

Even with a good historical relationship, arriving at common goals takes time and effort to resolve differences and build on consensus areas. As already indicated, hospitals must be sensitive to the physician's sense of lost security in giving up control of his or her medical practice. Therefore, the hospital must relate the physician's compensation to achievement of the goals described for the affiliation. Examples of these goals might include providing care to an indigent population in compliance with the hospital's mission, developing risk-sharing contracts with third-party payers, and achieving cost efficiencies through the consolidation of resources in providing ambulatory patient services. The hospital will need to do detailed research on the physicians' current income level from their practices.

The most frequent areas of goal conflict have to do with physician compensation, financial viability of the practice, or feasibility of changing hospital operations and practice operations to pursue risk-sharing contracts aggressively. Without mutually acceptable long-term and short-term goals, the relationship suffers.

Top-Level Leadership Involvement

Traditionally, physicians are the owners and managers of medical practices. In affiliation discussions, physicians expect top-level leaders of the hospital to become involved. There are several reasons for this expectation. For one thing, the development of trust between the parties requires visible commitment of hospital leaders—that is, through their presence at meetings—so that physicians are convinced an affiliated group practice is an important project for the hospital.

Another reason for hospital leader involvement is the substantial financial commitment the hospital is making to the joint effort. The hospital CEO and board representatives must be involved in planning and negotiations. To do this effectively, they must understand the group practice operations and the impact an affiliation will have on the hospital. Otherwise, internal conflict and implementation failure are imminent.

Finally, because an affiliated group practice usually affects only a few members of the medical staff, the satisfaction of knowing that top-level leaders are committed to the venture is crucial. It is a clear signal for the rest of the medical staff, one that will gain their acceptance of this project.

Governance and Control

Given a positive relationship between the hospital and physicians, the mutual commitment to the goals and objectives of an affiliated group practice, and involvement of top-level hospital leaders, issues related to the governance and control of the new entity can be addressed more easily. Physicians look to physicians for leadership, particularly in the clinical aspects of medical practice. Thus, an affiliated group practice must grant physicians authority over this aspect of the practice.

The selection of physician leaders is a difficult task. Success in operating a small group or solo practice does not automatically translate into strong leadership for a group practice. The economy and self-reliance so important in a solo practice may prove ineffective in working to develop consensus among a group of physicians. At the least, a physician leader should have the following attributes:

- An understanding and commitment to the strategies and goals of the group practice
- The respect of physicians in the group, both as a clinician and a manager
- The ability to work within a larger organization

The physician leader will need to focus on integrating physicians into the group practice operations. This focus will include not only developing clinical protocols that are acceptable and appropriate for all physicians, but also working with physicians individually and as a group to resolve issues such as call schedule, physician income distribution, space allocation, utilization of ancillary personnel, and medical records protocol. It is important that strong administrative leaders work with the physician leaders. Just as physicians need to have support when integrating into a group practice (support that can most effectively be provided through a physician leader), nonphysician personnel will also need support. Additionally, it is crucial that the administrative leader working with the physician leader be dedicated to the group practice so that the physician and administrator can work effectively as a team in developing a strong hospital-affiliated group practice.

☐ Planning and Negotiation

An important task of the planning process is to develop a *realistic business plan* for the venture. The plan should include the requirements for capital to purchase existing practice assets or develop new practice sites, as well as funding needed for the start-up operations of the affiliated group practice. Anticipated growth of the practice over a three-to-five-year period should be incorporated into the plan. A thorough understanding of the financial implications of an affiliated group practice is an important element in negotiating final agreements and establishing appropriate structures.

Negotiations should begin following agreement on the mutual benefit of this venture, its goals and objectives, and the financial requirements. Details of key elements of negotiation were discussed in earlier chapters and in the case studies but are briefly revisited in the following subsections.

Practice Purchase Price

The major components of a practice purchase price are detailed in chapter 4. Third-party appraisals and valuations help parties reach agreement on the sale price. The legal implications of a hospital's purchase of an existing practice must be considered in negotiating that price.

Physician Compensation

A competitive compensation structure, including incentives, motivates physicians to develop appropriate practice patterns. The following list presents important elements in a compensation package:

- Physician's current income (during start-up period only)
- Incomes for physicians in similar specialties in the market area and nationally
- Financial results of the affiliated group practice
- Patient volume or procedure productivity of the individual physician
- Capitated patient enrollment (where applicable)
- Factors directed at changing practice patterns (in highly capitated markets) such as patient satisfaction, wait time for patient appointments, utilization of resources, physician participation in group practice efforts to change practice patterns, and so forth

Balance must be reached between the physicians' expected compensation and the actual financial results of the affiliated group practice. To gain physicians' trust, it may be necessary to guarantee an initial period of income that closely approximates their current income. However, negotiations initially should include transition of compensations to relate more directly to the goals and objectives of the affiliated group.

Control

It is generally accepted that physicians need to control the clinical aspects of a medical practice, a need that is secured when medical staff leadership and committee structures are made up of physicians. However, the tradition of physician autonomy must be balanced against the hospital's need for control over its very large investment in developing an affiliated group practice. Control issues include the following:

- *Ownership of the medical practice:* Many hospital–group practice affiliations leave ownership of the medical practice with the physicians while the hard assets and management resources are owned by the hospital; others develop structures so that practice ownership is shared; still others, out of consideration for corporate practice of medicine laws, develop the structure in a way such that the hospital owns the practice. The major concern in assigning ownership is retention of physician loyalty to the hospital if practice ownership remains with physicians. A significant portion of the purchase price is embedded in the value of intangible practice assets. If physicians retain ownership they can receive payment for their practice as they retire from the group and new physicians buy into the practice. If the practice is purchased by the hospital, there will be no buyout when the physicians retire.
- *Physician compensation:* Physician compensation is complicated whenever the group is made up of physicians from a number of different specialties. Traditionally conflict has surrounded income distribution between primary care and specialist physicians. This conflict will be compounded as capitated revenue takes hold. One solution is to create a professional corporation to employ the physicians and to develop physician compensation to the group as a whole. This way, owners of the professional corporation determine what individual physicians will be paid. This leaves control of this issue in the physician's hands, with the hospital involved in developing overall compensation for professional services in negotiations with the physician-owned corporation.
- *Practice operations:* If the hospital is providing management resources and services to a physician-owned practice, shared control is accomplished through negotiating these service contracts. If physicians are employees of the hospital, a management committee, including physician representatives, should be established.

☐ Leadership, Management, and Flexibility

Successful implementation of an affiliated entity depends on several major issues related to leadership style and flexibility of the group practice systems and operations, including:

- *Practice management expertise:* The differences between medical practice operations and hospital operations already have been discussed. The difficulty with applying hospital management expertise in a group practice setting is reflected in several of the case studies. A successful group practice must have strong and experienced managers with group practice experience. Ability to empathize with physicians, understand physician billing systems, deal with capitated revenue distribution, and address other unique aspects of practice management are leadership requisites.
- *Leadership commitment to change:* An affiliated group practice will have a major impact on the long-term strategies of a hospital and the physicians involved in the group practice. They must be committed to the changes required to effect integration of these two business entities and to deal with the changing health care delivery and reimbursement environment.

    Much has been said about the changes required in physician practices, with preventive care and utilization control cited often. Hospitals must recognize, however, the departmental changes required to support a medical practice, as well as the effective utilization of the hospital's resources. Without strong leadership, this is impossible.

Leaders also must monitor their facility's environment in an attempt to determine the appropriate time for changes. It is difficult for physicians to change practice patterns to comply with capitated reimbursement when the majority of their reimbursement is through fee for service.

• *Group practice growth:* The factors leading to the growth of medical group practices have been highlighted throughout this text. The case studies indicate a significant growth in the number of physicians involved in a group practice following an affiliation with a hospital. Specific examples of growth are shown in table 13-2.

Initial participation in an affiliated group practice may be limited to the members of an existing group or to those physicians who recognize the importance of the group practice on their continued success and who are able to develop mutual goals with the hospital. Following implementation of an affiliated group practice and its successful operation, many additional physicians may be willing to join the group.

Therefore an affiliated group practice may well exceed the number of physicians anticipated in its planning. The group must be flexible in dealing with this situation, both in responding to the financial requirements of expansion, as well as maintaining a balance between successful implementation of group practice systems and the opportunity to increase the number of physicians.

• *Changing environment:* Changes in the local environment can create the need for flexibility in an affiliated group practice. Changes in competitor activity or in the reimbursement structure for health care in the community are environmental changes that can affect an affiliated group practice. Hospital leaders and members of an affiliated group practice must understand that in a changing environment, those systems and structures that are put in place during implementation may need to be modified. A rapid increase in capitated reimbursement may require modification of physician compensation. Increased competition from other integrated delivery systems may require rapid expansion of the group.

Table 13-2. Physician Growth in Group Practices

Institution	Number of Physicians during the Year That Affiliated Group Practice Operations Began	Number of Physicians as of December 1993
Midwest Medical Center	2 (1990)	12
Mercy Medical Foundation Sacramento, CA	62 (1990)	117
Good Samaritan San Jose, CA	18 (1992)	41
Millard Fillmore Buffalo, NY	1 (1986)	20
Mercy Hospital Pittsburgh, PA	3 (1986)	10
St. Luke's Saginaw, MI	1 (1990)	3
Monroe Clinic Monroe, WI	41 (1992)	51

If hospital leaders and physicians have successfully completed development of mutual goals and objectives, the strong leadership and flexibility required to adapt the affiliated group practice to internal and external demands will be in place. Group leaders must ensure that focus remains on long-term strategies and that changes in current operations be made when necessary.

□ Conclusion

The development of a hospital-affiliated group practice requires strong commitment on the part of the hospital and physicians. Trust, mutual motivations, and goals and objectives must be in sync prior to implementation.

Successful affiliations are significant investments of time and resources for both parties. Failure to address areas of potential conflict in goals will compromise implementation and jeopardize the venture.

It is impossible to ensure that all aspects of an affiliated group practice will be addressed in the planning and implementation stages. Flexibility in practice operations are essential to long-term success.

Despite the complexities and costs of developing an affiliated group practice, such an entity appears to be a viable vehicle for hospitals and physicians in a changing health care environment. With appropriate planning, negotiation, and flexibility following implementation, an affiliated group practice can lead to provision of top-quality health for a community.

Index

Abuse. *See* Fraud and abuse
Accounting
    accrual, 72
    cash, 72
Accounts receivable, value assigned to, 65
Accrual accounting, 72
Active investor, 86
Affiliation process, 15–16, 20
    implementation stage in, 29
    initial discussions stage in, 20–22
    motivations for, 109
    negotiation and issue resolution stage in, 28–29
    preliminary planning stage in, 16–20
    reevaluation stage in, 27–28
    research and detailed planning stage in, 22–27
    structure of, 109
Ambulatory surgery centers, investment interest safe harbors for, 85–86
American Medical Association, 67
Americans with Disabilities Act (ADA), and due diligence, 26
Ancillary services, 74
    group practice options in, 74
    in-office, 89–90
    integrated relationship options in, 74–75
    options for allocating revenues of, 74
Anticipation, principle of, 66
Antitrust issues, 99–100
    affiliation between physician group practice and hospital in, 100–101
    combined group practices in, 100
    safety zones in, 101–2
Arizona v. Maricopa County Medical Society, 101
Assets, hard, 65, 67
Autonomy, as obstacle to hospital–physician collaboration, 7–8

Blended industry rule-of-thumb method, 66, 68
Bona fide employment relationships, Stark Bill exception for, 91
Book value, 65
Bottom-line compensation, 71
Business enterprise value, 65
Business issues
    control and decision making in, 77, 78–79
    critical cost factors in, 75–76

due diligence in, 26
financial terms between parties in, 63–75
leadership in, 77, 80
negotiation and resolution of, 28
planning in affiliation process in, 24–25
political issues in, 76
Business options
    primary care versus multispecialty group, 60
    specialty networks in, 61
Buy-in arrangements in group practice, 5–6, 9

California Medical Association (CMA), 77
Capitalization. *See also* Cost and capitalization
    of excess earnings approach, 66
    full, 71–72
Capital needs
    in group practice, 5
    influence of on integration levels, 34
Captive professional corporations, 18
Case studies
    community need in, 208
    competition in, 208
    control in, 215
    criteria for, 109–10
    elements in, 111
    environment in, 208–10
    existing group practices in, 208–9
    flexibility in, 215–17
    goals and objectives in, 210–11, 213
    governance and control in, 213–14
    historical relationship in, 212
    hospital motivations in, 210–11
    leadership in, 213, 215–17
    managed care penetration in, 209–10
    management in, 215–17
    physician compensation in, 214
    physician motivations in, 211
    planning and negotiation in, 214–15
    practice purchase price in, 214
    relationship between hospitals and physicians in, 211–14
Cash accounting, 72
Center of excellence, 61
Clayton Act, 100
Cleveland Clinic, 57, 109
Clinical issues and due diligence, 26–27
Clinical Laboratory Improvement Amendments (CLIA) and due diligence, 26

Clinton, Bill, and health care reform, 34, 93–94
Closed-panel physician–hospital organization, 40–41
Codependence of separate entities, 32
Collaboration, 3–4
    assessing options for, 18–19
    candidates for, 20
    strategic, 17
    tactical, 17–18
Combined group practice, antitrust and market considerations for, 100
Community benefit test, 95–96
Community need, 208
Comparable sale method, 66–67
Compensation. *See* Employee compensation; Physician compensation
Competition, 208
    and growth of managed care, 1–2
    influence of on integration levels, 34
Conditional management service organization, 45
Contingency issues, negotiation and resolution of, 28–29
Control, 213–15
    and decision making, 77, 78
    in group practice, 8–9
Controlled group rules, 103
Corporate practice of medicine, 98
    minimizing risk of law violations in, 98–99
Cost and capitalization. *See also* Capitalization
    in direct physician employment model, 55–56
    in foundation model, 49
    in management service organization model, 46
    in physician equity model, 58–59
    in physician–hospital organization model, 38
    in trust/professional corporation model, 52–53
Cost of operations and infrastructure, 75
Coverage test, 103
Credentialing criteria in physician–hospital organization (PHO), 40
Critical cost factors, 75–76

Daughters of Charity Health System (St. Louis), 58
Decision making and control, 77, 78

(continued on next page)

Index

Monroe Clinic/St. Clare Hospital
(continued)
  ancillary services, 204
  employee integration, 203–4
  financing, 204, 205
  physician compensation, 204
  practice valuation, 202–3
  planning process, 200
    awareness and issues identification, 200
    benefits of consolidation, 201
    issues resolution, 201
    planning results, 201–2
    presentation of plan, 202, 203
Mullikin Medical Group, 56, 57, 58, 59
Multispecialty group versus primary care, 60
Mutual funds, Stark Bill exceptions for, 90

Negotiation and issue resolution in affiliation process, 28–29
Nondiscrimination tests, 102–3
Nonprofit corporation, and income taxation, 95

Obstacles to hospital–physician integration process, 7–8
Ochsner Clinic, 57
Office of Inspector General (OIG), 84
Office space, Stark Bill exception for rental of, 90–91
Omnibus Budget Reconciliation Act (1993), 88–89
One-purpose test, 84
Open panel, 39–40
Operational standards, establishment of, 29
Operational test for tax-exempt status, 95–96
Organizational assessment, 27
Organizational options. *See also* Legal issues
  direct physician employment model, 54–57
  foundation model, 47–51
  hospital ownership of practice site and assets model, 42–43
  management service organization model, 43–44
  physician equity model, 57–60
  physician–hospital organization model, 36–42
  practice enhancement service model, 35–36
  service bureau model, 35–36
  trust/professional corporation model, 51–54
Organizational test for tax-exempt status, 95
Ownership, in group practice, 8–9

Pacific Physician Services, 57, 59
Participation test, 103
Patient advocacy, as obstacle to hospital–physician collaboration, 8
Payout arrangements in group practice, 9
Personal relationships, influence of on integration levels, 33
Personal service, safe harbor for, 87
Personal service contracts, Stark Bill exception for, 91

Physician compensation, 68–69, 214. *See also* Employee compensation
  bonuses, 70
  bottom line, 71
  control of, 73
  in direct physician employment model, 56
  employee benefit plans in, 72
  in foundation model, 49–50
  full capitation, 71–72
  in group practice, 9
  managed care pools/withholds, 71
  other compensation factors, 72
  in physician equity model, 59
  and private inurement, 94–95
  production-based, 71
  quality-based incentives, 70
  salary, 70
  summary of mechanisms, 69
Physician defection, in foundation model, 50
Physician equity organizational model, 57–58
  capabilities and limitations of, 60
  control in, 59
  cost and capitalization in, 58–59
  operations in, 59
  other issues in, 59–60
  physician compensation in, 59
  structure of, 58
Physician–hospital organization (PHO), 18, 32, 36–37. *See also* Group practice
  capabilities and limitations of, 41–42
  closed-panel, 38, 40–41
  cost and capitalization in, 38
  functions of, 37–38
  open-panel, 38–40
  other issues in, 41
  participation in, 38–39
  physician credentialing criteria in, 39–40
  planning for, 37
  structure of, 39
Physician integration, levels of, 69
Physician network joint ventures, antitrust safety zone for, 101–2
Physician organization, 40
Physicians
  autonomy of, 33
  classification of as specialists versus primary care, 2
  influence of needs on integration levels, 33
  mind-set of, as obstacle to hospital–physician collaboration, 7–8
  needs of, and influence on integration levels, 33
  participation of in managed care contracting, 2
  payments by, for items and services, 93
  perspective on collaboration with hospital, 5–7, 211–14
  recruitment and retention of, and influence on integration levels, 34
  Stark Bill exception for payments by, 93
Physician self-referrals, 88
  Stark Bill exceptions, 88–94
    for hospital ownership, 90
    for in-office ancillary services, 89–90
    for ownership in publicly traded securities and mutual funds, 90

for physician services, 89
for prepaid plans, 90
for rental of office space and equipment, 90–91
for rural providers, 90
Physician services, Stark Bill exception for, 89
Planning
  preliminary, 16–20
  strategic, 23–24
Political issues, 76
Practice
  hospital ownership of site and assets, 42–43
  purchase versus equity swap, 53
  safe harbor for sale of, 87
Practice enhancement services, 35–36
Practice valuation and purchase, 63–64, 68, 214
  accounts receivable in, 65
  allocation of value in, 68
  framework for, 67
  hard assets in, 65
  hospital perspective of, 64
  intangibles in, 65–68
  other considerations in, 68
  physician perspective of, 64
  valuation methods in, 64–68
Preferred provider organization (PPO), 88, 101
  percentage of physicians likely to contract with, 2
Preliminary planning, 16–20
Prepaid plans, Stark Bill exception for, 90
Primary care
  demand for, 2
  focus on, 4
  versus multispecialty groups, 60
Primary care center development. *See* Millard Fillmore Hospital System
Private inurement and tax-exempt status, 94–95
Problem identification by exploratory task force, 22
Production-based physician compensation, 71
Professional corporation. *See* Trust/professional corporation organizational model
Professional services, inurement risks with compensation for, 95

Rabbi trusts, 102
Recruitment
  alternate support scenarios, 6
  and hospital–physician collaboration, 5
Reevaluation stage in affiliation process, 27–28
Regulatory compliance issues and due diligence, 26
Remuneration, Stark Bill exception for unrelated, 92
Replacement value, 65
Research and detailed planning in affiliation process, 22–27
Resources, influence on integration levels, 34
Retirement plans, 102
Revenue guarantee, 75
Rule-of-reason analysis, 100

Additional Books of Interest

**Community Health Information Networks: Creating the
Health Care Data Highway**
edited by Ralph T. Wakerly and First Consulting Group

This book focuses on the concepts, approaches, and trends in information technology that will have lasting value to readers. Divided into two parts, the book covers both the strategic issues of interest to senior executives and the practical hands-on information needed by the technical experts. Whether read from cover to cover, or used as a handy reference for specific issues, *Community Health Information Networks* will prove very useful.
Catalog No. E99-093104 (must be included when ordering)
1994. 200 pages, 36 figures, 15 tables, glossary.
$56.00 (AHA members, $45.00)

**The Physician–Computer Connection: A Practical Guide
to Physician Involvement in Hospital Information Systems**
by William F. Bria II, M.D., and Richard L. Rydell

This well-written book shows hospital administrators and information systems professionals how to enlist physicians in the selection, design, and implementation of patient care information systems (PCIS) and how to overcome physician resistance to using computer systems in their day-to-day clinical decision making and patient care activities. Readers will learn how to break down the barriers that often discourage physicians from using computer systems.
Catalog No. E99-093102 (must be included when ordering)
1992. 110 pages, 6 figures.
$37.50 (AHA members, $29.95)

Medical Staff Credentialing: A Practical Guide
by Fay A. Rozovsky, J.D., Lorne E. Rozovsky, LL.B., and Linda M. Harpster, J.D.

Medical Staff Credentialing is designed for administrators and physicians who are either directly involved in the credentialing process or need to know how that process works. The book focuses on the basic practical problems of determining whether, and to what extent, a physician will be permitted to practice within the hospital. It covers the credentialing process, from initial application and clinical privilege delineation, through periodic reassessment, to reappointment and reprivileging.
Catalog No. E99-145102 (must be included when ordering)
1993. 132 pages, 8 figures.
$49.00 (AHA members, $39.00)

To order, call TOLL FREE
1-800-AHA-2626